NATIVE AMERICAN

HERBALISM
ENCYCLOPEDIA

The forgotten secrets of medicinal
plants & their uses for healing

TAMAYA KAWISENHAWE

This tool does not provide medical advice It is intended for informational purposes only. It is not a substitute for professional medical advice, diagnosis or treatment. Never ignore professional medical advice in seeking treatment because of something you have read on the WebMD Site. If you think you may have a medical emergency, immediately call your doctor or dial 911.

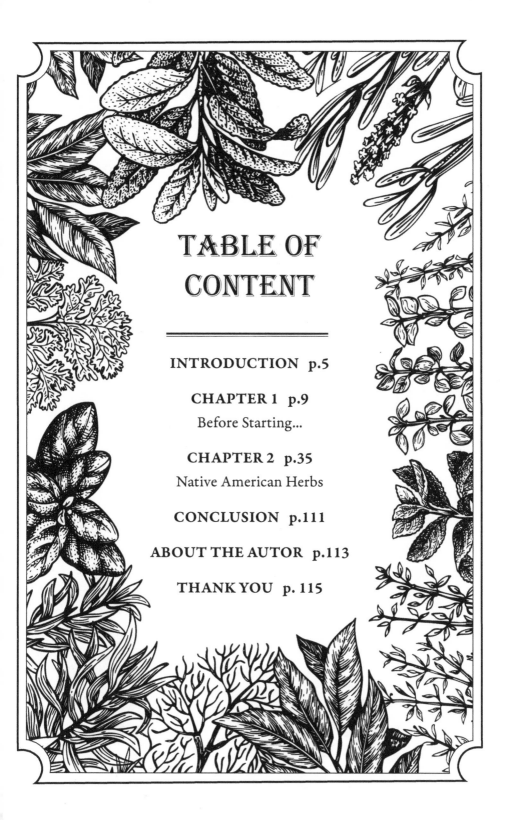

TABLE OF CONTENT

INTRODUCTION

The theory that underlies all medicinal, physical, and spiritual Native American healing therapies is quite basic. People must learn to live in peace with the world around them in order to live healthily. In a way, the first ecologists were Native Americans. They wanted their relationship with Mother Earth to be as harmonious as possible, and they believed that eternal stability, which was necessary for good health, would only be accomplished when they existed in harmony with the world. In recent years, it has been apparent that they were on to something. Analysis has found that our mental wellbeing influences physical fitness tremendously.

Lewis Mehl-Madrona, M.D., Medical Director of the Centre for Complementary Medicine at the University of Pittsburgh Medical

"If we are in peace with the world and the people around us, our cells are in equilibrium inside us...Amid the difficulties she sent her way, the Native Americans sought ways of living in peace with Mother Earth." *

They committed themselves to keep all facets of their world in the highest esteem, including wild animals and poor weather. For example, when they killed a bear, they made a necklace with their teeth, worn by a warrior to honour the bravery and strength of the beast. They have often left presents such as small tobacco pouches after every good hunt to express their heartfelt thanks to Mother Earth. In the same way, they treated trees. They still did so with deep reverence, whether they cultivated plants for Medicine or fruit. They claimed that it was their way of expressing appreciation for the kindness of the Supreme Spirit, which was responsible for all living things. They claimed that a refusal to live in accordance with Mother Nature would have dire repercussions, for example, by not giving adequate thanks for good hunts and harvests. An Indian who hunted animals or gathered herbs would always sing the requisite songs or prayers or give tobacco offerings to the spirits of the animals or plants, according to one scholar, "as failure to do so could lead to sickness or bad luck." Only a few decades ago, modern ears sounded odd about this mystical approach to nature and the environment. Americans also began to see the wisdom of the holistic approach, though. The common expression "what goes around comes around" reflects how much we have come to accept the Native American way of life and respect it.

The wellness traditions and values of Native American tribes are related to Native American Medicine. Although some of these traditions exist today in some tribes, this paper looks at the issue from a historical point of view, mainly concentrating on historical sources as opposed to current traditions.

In many Native American tribes, healthcare has historically focused on the principle of harmony in every area of life. It was believed that physical, cultural, emotional, and environmental components all played a role in the wellbeing of the participant and the community. Usually, diseases are not due to physical disease alone, but rather an inconsistency in any or more of these components. As a result, many tribes claimed that both natural and spiritual causes could be the result of disease, and their medicine activities were meant to cope with both.

The tradition of Native American Medicine dates back thousands of years, but pre-European evidence of these rituals is almost non-existent since most tribes never produced a written language. Before Europeans started to gather in the 16th century in continental America, no outsiders had ever been able to capture these customs.

Furthermore, most Native American medicine practitioners at the time had no desire to share their expertise with outsiders, claiming that such experience was sacred. The adaptable, variable existence of Native American herbalism (discussed further down under Medicine) made it so that no encyclopedic medicinal works could be conveniently published to further exacerbate the matter. At that very moment, past documents of anyone's healthcare profession serve as a snapshot of an individual tribe and do not generally represent Native American Medicine as a whole. However, to recognize popular patterns and customs, these individual instances can nevertheless be observed.

The advances in medical research have had a huge effect on our lives, no doubt. Individuals enjoy fuller, happier lives than ever before. Any of the advantages of modern drugs, however, can be offset by their costs. Modern medications are pricey, not only in billions but in terms of our long-term wellbeing, maybe. That's how most operate by causing the body to answer in some ways, as powerful as medications can be, rather than by relying on the body's own natural healing forces. The body may be placed in a passive, reliant, and gradually impaired state by using medications. Remember what happens with an illness when you get it. Taking an antibiotic, which destroys the bacteria that make you sick, is the latest solution. This is a rational solution in the short term, but every day, the body is exposed to billions of bacteria. It is a losing cause in the long run. Antibiotics are just temporary protection, although essential for battling certain infections. They don't help the body improve its own defences and avoid new pathogens.
A completely new approach was taken by aboriginal healers. In their opinion, the better solutions were those that enabled the body to take care of itself instead of just offering immediate assistance. They also strongly believed in a spiritual aspect of healing that reinforced the body as well as the mind and emotions through meditation, imagination, and a number of healing rituals, making a recovery much simpler. Today, this mind-body relation is being embraced by a growing number of established practitioners. It took hundreds of years, but Native Americans' wisdom and expertise are now on the cutting edge of mainstream medical treatment.

In reality, the recent increase in "alternative" methods of healing and the use of therapeutic prayer recalls Native American methods: herbs and other so-called "natural" medicines, imagination, meditation, and more. Many individuals are shocked to discover how experienced Native Americans actually were. Mostly, in a somewhat small way, culture portrays these knowledgeable, insightful persons. Although it is accurate that Native Americans were skilled hunters, instrument-makers, and warriors, their talents were larger than that. None has been said of their remarkable skills as healers until recently. Native Americans were well-known among the early colonists for supposedly impressive curing abilities, but historians documented little of these tales, possibly owing to ethnic bias and the assumption that "savages" were Native Americans. However, reports of Native American medical prowess began to circulate by word of mouth and were reported in colonial diaries and journals. Still, we will read first-hand accounts of what the Native Americans were able to do from the early settlers.

Before Starting...

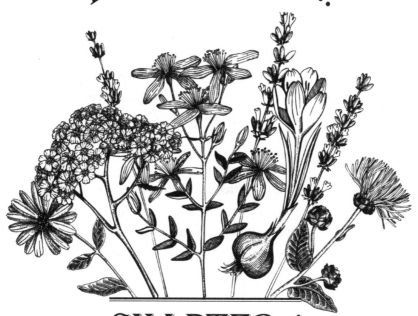

CHAPTER 1

Herbalism usually refers to traditional medicinal practice based on the use of plants and plant extracts. Herbalism is also known as phototherapy. In this chapter, we will be discussing wildcrafting, growing, and storage of herbs for Herbalism.

1.1 WILDCRAFTING

The process of collecting plants from their natural environment for nutritional or therapeutic purposes is wildcrafting. (The term 'foraging' is sometimes used, but they are synonymous, for grain and 'wildcrafting' for herbal medicines). Wildcrafted herbs can be used in a number of medicines, including tinctures, herbal salves, and infusions, and when handled mindfully, you can enjoy all the benefits of wild herbal medicines without upsetting the environment.

Wildcrafting Benefits

Wild plants, since they come from richer terrain, mostly in relatively undisturbed meadows and forests, are more potent and nutrient-dense than their monoculture counterparts. Commercial farms also have depleted soil or feed isolated nutrients to the plants only. It is a perfect way to experience the outdoors as well. For a relaxing expedition, you should bring a mate. And there are many easy herbal remedies you can make with your harvest of wild plants when you return home.

WILDCRAFTING HERBS WILL HELP YOUR EFFORTS TO:

Eat foods that are nutrient-dense
Reduce reliance on imported medicines and food
Decrease reliance on Major Agro
Experience and enjoy nature

With natural tonics & remedies, keep yourself healthy! At the same time, you can also bring family and friends along and build a community.

What to bring when you're going wildcrafting:

You don't really need a lot of equipment, but there are a few essentials that can really make your journey a smooth one. You're going to need something mostly to bring your harvest in, and you may need some instruments to distinguish the plants from the forest.

For short journeys, baskets are great, and for longer ones, big paper bags are great. Don't store herbs in plastic because they can decompose quickly in the sun. You would need something for slicing, digging and snipping, depending on what you want to harvest. If you're digging roots, you'll want a trowel, and if you have to hack bark or roots, bring a decent knife, and some kitchen shears or scissors for snipping greenery or flowers.

For all kinds of wildcrafting and gardening duties, I love this Hori digging knife. It has one smooth blade and one serrated blade and it is angled so that it acts as a knife and a trowel. A vegetable brush is another handy tool to clean roots with, to reduce the dirt you take with you. Carry a paintbrush instead of a crop brush if you're picking mushrooms to avoid destroying them.

1.2. SITE SELECTION

Obtaining permission: On BLM property, if you receive limited sums, a free use permit can be received for a low fee. The U.S. Both Forest Service and BLM will warn you that there is no picking (a) in or near campgrounds or picnic areas; (b) some trails less than 200 feet away; and (c) on the side of the lane.

1. Keep away from downwind runoff, roadsides (at least 50 feet), electric high-voltage cables (may cause mutations), lawn and public park fertilizers, downstream mines or agribusiness, near parking lots, and even spray areas. Routine spraying is used by several BLM and Forest Service areas. This also refers to private property, where you would need to worry about herbicides and pesticides.

2. A reckless wildcrafter will seriously alter a rocky hillside or stream-side habitat using discretion in vulnerable ecosystems.

1.3. GROWING AND PROPAGATION TECHNIQUES

1. Using proper techniques for wild crafts can ensure minimal effects, improve harvest yields, and help to provide wildlife with plant food. Year after year, do not harvest the same stand but tend the field as needed. Techniques used for "gardening" include thinning, root separation, top pinching, and protection of a wide variety of grandparent plants to seed and protect young plants.

2. Be mindful of conditions contributing to erosion. Replant or disperse seeds if digging roots and close gaps. Be conscious of stands on the hillside, add vegetation and soil around areas cleared. It could be appropriate to gather foliage from surrounding collected plants and scatter it around. Wearing hard-soled shoes can inflict irreparable harm to fragile hillside ecosystems.

3. Don't pull the roots while extracting the leaves. Root yields, as well as foliage, can be improved by flower pruning of some species.

4. Allow seasonal findings on areas produced by wildlife. Be mindful of your harvested stands and check the various cycles of growth. This will measure the true effect on the Environment. (An established wild crafter in the northwest has found that a stable population would rise by around 30% a year once it enters stasis. Anything less than this may be called degenerative.)

1.4. SUGGESTED GATHERING TIMES

1. Aerial or above-ground parts: from 6 to 10 a.m. in the mornings, just until they wilt in the light. Some are stronger just before flowering when collecting leaves.

2. You should be able to see the bud's colour by picking most flowers only before they are starting to bloom. Around or after the full moon is the typical moon period for collecting aerial parts.

3. **Roots:** Harvest after seeding; early in the morning, if possible, before the sun reaches. Biennials: harvest in the first year's fall or the second year's season. A new moon is a conventional period.

4. **Barks:** In the spring or autumn, harvest. Don't strip ever. Take a whole crop. In dense cities, tree thinning is acceptable, but the healthiest looking trees still leave. Be mindful of potentially leaving the tree vulnerable to fungal rot if you take only from the small branches. The inner bark, or cambium, is the most active bark of many, for pollarding, leaving short trunks and low stumps for coppicing. This will supply a continuous production. The typical bark process is three-quarters of the waning light.

5. **Saps & Pitches:** Late winter or early spring harvest.

6. **Seed & Fruit:** Harvest when ripe, with some variations, such as oranges, unripe pods of scarlet beans, etc.

1.5. DRYING

1. Dry most plants in shaded, well-ventilated areas; avoid wire screens and newspaper print. Research which plants dry better in the sun.

2. Don't wash the flowers or plants. Shake them to clear off pests and ashes. Where amounts are reasonable, tie bundles with diameters of 1 1/2 inches or less at the stems' base. They can also be loosely dispersed to dry on windows.

3. Barks: If possible, peel the outer bark off. It's called tossing here.

4. Roots: Spread out or loop them. Usually, rinsing won't dissolve soil particles. As well as hand brushing, particularly with clay, a pressure hose is often needed. For broad, heavy roots without aromatic properties, cut lengthwise.

5. When fragile, all plant components are dry. Pinch the hanging plants in the lower section. To see if the core is dry, cut a large sample root in half.

TO PRODUCE INFUSIONS OF HOT WATER

Leaves:
1 ounce per quart of water, 4 hours in hot water, securely sealed.
Tougher leaves need steeping for longer.

Flowers:
1 ounce per quart of water, in hot water for 2 hours.
Less time is needed for more delicate flowers.

Seeds:
1 ounce per pint of water, in hot water for 30 minutes.
Less time is required for more fragrant seeds such as fennel (15 minutes),
longer rose hips (3 to 4 hours).

Barks & Roots:
1 ounce per pint of water, in hot water for 8 hours.
Less (1 to 2 hours) for certain barks,
such as slippery elm.

1.6. STORAGE

1. Stop heat that is light and excessive and might kill aromatic properties and other important constituents. Food grade plastic bags or fiber barrels or other containers that emit oxygen and moisture are suitable to retain consistency and potency as long as possible while they are completely dry.

2. Mark with place and dates.

3. Broken or crushed herbs lose their worth more easily than uncut herbs, which are complete.

The Rocky Mountain Herbalists' Group has established approaches to conserving wild medicinal plant species. Deep feelings for the sanctity of the Environment and plant communities are the impetus for developing these methods. As a non-governmental group operating in a single bioregion, these techniques are structured to include informed self-interest and social coercion. These methods are available for use, modified, and implemented to their own unique needs by those in other bioregions.

The first move was to establish a series of rules to help harvesters grasp the core concepts of ethical wildlife crafting. With many experienced wildcrafters' feedback, these standards have been established and submitted to rigorous peer review. Instead of being hard and fast guidelines, they are built to compliment the ethical framework. For the wildcrafter to fill out and submit along with each shipment of herbs, a requirements sheet containing details on where and how a plant is grown, handled, and dried has been produced. This data offers customers the ability to learn about responsible wildlife crafting and explicitly help harvesters whose philosophies are in line with their own.

The next move was to establish a list of conscientious wild craftsmen and organic farmers for direct marketing. By placing herb buyers in line with the actual harvesters, the register was designed to promote good actions. This direct connection promotes an atmosphere of shared interest, helps improve quality management, and encourages wildcrafters to set rates that enhance sustainable harvesting practices and inspire them.

Manufacturers of herbal products are encouraged to use the list to integrate the values into their routine business activities. Wild crafters and organic farmers who are ecologically conscious are invited to send additional listings to the new register. The development of a bio-regional cooperative of wild craftsmen and organic farmers is a recent phase in this initiative.

The concept is to come together as a group to share information; encourage education among harvesters and growers; establish self-regulation systems by peer review; and meet demands at a price that promotes healthy, ecologically sound practices for ethically harvested and organically grown herbs. The co-op is a vehicle for participants to exchange knowledge about plant growth patterns, harvesting procedures, methods of propagation and production, and alternatives to over-harvesting. A list of native plants that are threatened, threatened, over-cultivated, or illegally cultivated is being established, and restrictions are set to ensure species' survival by peer consensus.

This knowledge can be shared in a newsletter with other wildcrafters, bio-regional co-ops, and customers. It is also possible to establish a seed sharing scheme so that regions can be re-seeded for potential use. For the co-op, to ensure that some areas are not overused and that other regions are left behind to regenerate, participants will be able to exchange knowledge on harvesting regions. The cooperative aims to create a system that can be used to direct each other and develop personal honesty. In order to protect areas from forestry, construction, and agriculture, the co-op may also be seen as a forum for citizens to work together as activists. We would like to see the development of an annual meeting where wild craftsmen can meet, exchange data, reinforce the network, and become a prominent, active member of the herbal culture.

There is an urgency for those who hear the sound of the Earth weeping, Herbalist or not, to do something to respond. This is a start to secure and help this tiny portion of the planet survive. The Rocky Mountain Herbalists' Alliance insists that we must be careful not to kill wild plant species or the wild places where they live either directly through our own acts or implicitly through our implicit agreement. To do this, we need to take precautions to put long-term survival at the grassroots and corporate level before short-term gain. If we take a stand together and stick to ethical values, those who disregard the plants will either change their processing methods or vanish from the sector. In this way, we seek to undo the harm done by our forebears, retain our own sacred faith in the World, and give our descendants the gift of respect for life seen on stable and prosperous earth.

1.7. HERBAL PREPARATIONS: MAKING INFUSIONS AND DECOCTIONS

An infusion is made by immersing an herb in either cold or hot (not boiling) water. The stream, not drinking water, can be the purest you can find. It is safer to provide water from rainfall, good wells or streams, or bottled water. Herbs with potent volatile oils are better infused in cold water (those with a clear scent like essential oil or perfume). In warm water, some herbs perform well. Depending on the plant, they can be left for a period of time, from fifteen minutes to overnight, so that the water will consume the plant's basic elements. For the production of infusions and decoctions, glass or earthenware vessels are great. As they won't crack from fire, quart or pint canning jars are fine, and the screw cap prevents the nutrients from floating away in the steam.

An Example Of A Hot Infusion

This infusion is used because of its general nutritional properties, especially for menopausal women. For anyone weighing 130 to 160 pounds, the rule-of-thumb is to take an infusion of 16 ounces (2 cups) every day.

1. Mix together the dried, sliced, and sifted nettles, oat-straw, red clover, alfalfa, horsetail, and spearmint for one pound each.
2. Place one cup of the mixture in a quart pot, fill it with hot water, and screw on the lid.
3. Just quit overnight.
4. Strain the mixture in the morning to extract all the ingredients and then drink it for the next two days. As they tend to go poor, do not keep infusions for more than two days.

For herbs, which work differently in cold and hot water, cold infusions are preferable. Yarrow, for example, when cooked in hot water, can be very bitter, but when cooked in cold water, it is not bitter. Yarrow's aromatic components, and their associated antispasmodic properties, are soluble in cold water, while the herb's acidic components are not. Cool infusions are formulated the same way as hot infusions, but a time span unique to itself would need to be soaked in each herb. This can only be learned over time, while several herbal books on the market can offer advice. Prepared with hot water, decoctions can be far more potent than infusions. In three cups of water, the general procedure is to slowly take one ounce of herb and simmer slowly until the liquid decreases by half. Use just a bottle made of stainless steel or glass, never aluminium. Depending on the plant employed, the dosages will vary from a tablespoon to a cup. The decoctions should be kept refrigerated for a period of two days only.

Tincturing Herbs

A tincture for internal use is made by immersing a fresh or dry plant in either straight alcohol or an alcohol and water mixture. Plants produce a certain amount of water when young, naturally. A fresh herb, one part of an herb per two parts of alcohol, is put in 190-proof alcohol (95 percent alcohol). If you had three ounces (dry measure) of fresh yarrow, for example, it would be placed in a container of 190-proof alcohol with six ounces (liquid measure), Mason jars are really good. The cap is screwed on, and the tincture is kept out of the heat for two weeks. It is decanted at the end of the duration, and the herb is pressed onto a rag to extract as much moisture as possible. Alcohol sucks all the water it absorbs out of a plant. A combination of both water and alcohol would be the resultant tincture. While many herbalists do so with fresh herbs, I do not cut or chop them into small bits. They assume that the heavier the tincture, the greater the surface area that is subjected to the alcohol. The herbs like to be kept whole in my job. We seldom develop fresh tincture roots. We cut them into smaller pieces as we do so. We still leave as whole as we can while tincturing the above-ground plant stuff. Each person must learn what works best. Plants lose their natural moisture content when they mature. There are tables on the moisture content of many medicinal plants available. Michael Moore, from his Southwest School of Botanical Medicine, gives a strong one. Certain plants have almost nothing, such as myrrh gum, and others have plenty of water, such as mint. When you make a dry plant tincture, the amount of water that was present in the plant when it was fresh is added back into the mixture. Dried plants are typically tinctured at a five-to-one ratio; that is, five liquid pieces to one dried herb part. The Osha root, for example, contains 30 percent water by weight. You'd apply fifty ounces of liquid, 35 ounces of 95% alcohol, and 15 ounces of water to it if you had ten ounces of powdered Osha core. You don't want to use drinking water ever since freshwater is a must.

As a general rule, dried herbs are powdered as thinly as possible, often in a blender. Until they are required, it is best to store them whole. Again, the tincture is left for two weeks and then decanted, and the medicinal content is squeezed out of the oil. For new seeds, you will normally pull as many out as you put in. You get out as much as you can with dry stuff, specifically roots. As they shield the tincture's purity from the chemical deterioration that can result from sunlight, amber jars are useful for tincture preservation. So safe, several years will last for the tinctures. For dispensing, herbal tinctures should then be mixed together (though a few do not mix well). Many herbalists choose tinctures because of their long-lasting consistency and ease of dispensing. In several herbal texts, dosages for tinctures are included.

TINCTURE FORMULA FOR UPSET STOMACH AND NAUSEA

Ten millilitres each of yarrow, poleo mint (or peppermint), and betony
Place in a one-ounce amber bottle with dropper
Take 1/3 to 1/2 dropper as needed

Making Oil Infusions For Salves

The first part of making a salve is to transfer the plant's medicinal properties to an oil base. Then the oil is made thick and moderately hard by the addition of beeswax. To make an oil infusion of dried herbs, grind the herbs you wish to use into as fine a powder as possible. Place the ground herbs in a glass baking dish and cover with oil. Olive oil is a good choice. Stir the herbs to make sure they are well saturated with oil and then add enough oil to cover them by 1/2 to 1/4 inch. Cook them in the oven on low heat for eight hours (overnight). Some herbalists prefer to cook the herbs as long as ten days at 100 degrees. When ready, strain the herbs' oil by pressing in a strong cloth with a good weave. To make an oil infusion from fresh herbs, place the herbs in a mason jar, and cover them with just enough oil to make sure that no part of the plant is exposed to air. Let sit in the sun for two weeks. Then press the herbs through a cloth. Let the decanted oil sit. After a day, the water, naturally present in the herbs, will settle to the bottom. Pour off the oil and discard the water. Some herbalists prefer to start the oil infusion by letting the herb sit for 24 hours in just a bit of alcohol that has been poured over the leaves. They then add the oil and allow it to stand for two weeks. The water and alcohol remain behind when the oil is poured off.

1.8. USEFUL INFORMATION ABOUT HERBALISM

In many ways, you can learn about herbs. Teachers who exchange experiences and practical information are one of the best opportunities to understand. They will have keen insights into herbs and their applications. Find educators who follow the ancient methods of herbal medicine within your culture. Take a lesson or workshop, or work on a farm with plants. To receive insights on how to manage the plants, form a mentoring relationship. It is also important that the plants spend time with you. Pick a plant that grows in your yard or sit down with a cup of herbal tea outdoors.

What are you seeing?
What is it that smells like?
How does it make you feel when you drink
tea made from grass?

Your experience is incomplete until you've spent time feeling, hearing, smelling, and eating the herb. And then you may, of course, check the many books on herbs and Herbalism which are available. We are lucky to have access to books written years ago and to books written since then for centuries. They include multiple facets and factors of herbal medicine (such as astrology), and most agree on the plant should be used where and how each one is used. This expertise was derived from years of analysis, training, and practice. However, once in a while, you can find data that varies from what you have heard elsewhere in one source. With the diverse viewpoints they often discover when they study herbs, I try to find fun in my students' desperation. This is a positive thing, though! Each Herbalist gives a thorough account of his or her own experience with the herb and how it functions. This knowledge is the product of the Herbalist's interaction with the plant. For the same leaf, you might have a slightly different experience, and that is good. Several herbal practitioners can agree that when they are eaten, herbs have unique purposes. Herbs help remove waste from the body. If the body undergoes slow digestion or insufficient detoxification, herbs move the old to make room for the fresh. Herbs facilitate recovery. Their vitamins and minerals intake help the body to regenerate and recover normal structure and function. In the body, herbs increase overall energy. Herbs offer a reinforcement that helps cure and detoxify the body, which raises the vitality levels of everyday life.

This book is for the herbal lover, who is searching for a lot of data in one location at the outset. Many herbal books concentrate on particular herbs, medication, or herbal history, but I decided to write a book with a little bit of both, both from a conventional and a science point of view. I am a gatherer of knowledge as a herbalist and biochemist, and naturopathic practitioner. My effort to share some of what I have heard about herbs in this book. In a metaphysical, science, and conventional way, I hope its components can help you understand herbal medicine. I have given the knowledge that I hope will help you interpret this complex method from a holistic viewpoint by mixing together anatomy, plant definitions, and herbal therapy concepts to develop a clearer understanding of how and when to use plants as medicine.

Remember that traditional Herbalism is much more complicated than what is described in this book when you begin your herbal studies. Herbalism focuses on a broader basis that incorporates the principles of tissue conditions (excitement, depression, atrophy, stagnation, anxiety, relaxation), the four characteristics of the plant (hot, cold, dry, damp), the disposition of the consumer, and the vitality (the subtle energies). We may not even know how herbs work as medicine, but there are several philosophies. However, we know that they act to manage whole body processes in a systemic manner rather than a single symptom. They nourish and maintain equilibrium in the body such that disharmonious organs will return to full operation. As a plant is introduced into the body, at a cellular stage, it is recognized. The body recognizes the constituents of the plant and appears to understand how to break them down and bring them to function where they are needed. While herbs can be beneficial at many physiological dimensions and measures, they work first with the body to identify and care for the region in greatest need. We can also get imaginative with preparation, mixing different herbs into formulations that concentrate with a much greater aim.

Many herbs are rich in minerals that supply the body with the required healing components to promote cell regeneration, digestion, digestion, and heart functionality. After herbs are administered to demonstrate their efficacy, we may clinically evaluate their physiological function. List some cases. Ginger produces very strong compounds called gingerols, which are anti-inflammatory. Several clinical trials involving patients with arthritis showed that ginger extracts influenced the inflammatory mechanism at the cellular level to alleviate discomfort and inflammation. Blood cell counts assessed following immune-stimulating herb administration indicate elevated amounts of white cells. Good improvements in cellular structure have been seen by biopsies obtained during herbal administration. Modern medicine has done an outstanding job in isolating plants and body elements, but the complex concepts in holism and structural harmony are seriously absent. Be mindful of the entire structure rather than the particular parts or signs, whether you are contemplating a plant or the body.

When you use herbs, think in a holistic way about the whole plant and how it can affect the body. Meadowsweet tea, for instance, is often used to cure problems with the stomach and can be especially effective for children with diarrhoea. Salicylic acid, which is an essential ingredient in aspirin, is one constituent (a chemically active portion within the herb) of meadowsweet. If salicylic acid is swallowed in an isolated way, the stomach wall can become irritated. But meadowsweet contains antioxidants called polyphenols, in addition to salicylic acid, that protect the stomach wall. This ensures that the desired behaviour of pain relief is provided by meadowsweet without the side effect of stomach discomfort.

I never see a patient in my office who is facing a problem in isolation. It is possible that other systems or organs are still failing when one system or organ is struggling. We ought to remember some significant points when we use herbs when we incorporate this way of thought to heal the body from a holistic viewpoint. Identify the trigger and handle it. While acute cases, such as burns, can often be rapidly soothed with herbs, study and the fostering of equilibrium within all body systems are necessary for long-standing disharmony. Look at the body as a whole. What physical pain do you consider normal? What signs have you endured for so long that they are almost no longer noticed by you? We may become detached from what is happening in our bodies and the symptoms and signals of pain in the hustle and bustle of our busy lives. Trust in nature's strength. Take a look around, and you can find that everywhere there are medicinal plants. Many plants that thrive in some regions are unique to the treatment of that region's diseases. For example, where I live in the Pacific Northwest, rosemary and cedar plants grow in abundance.

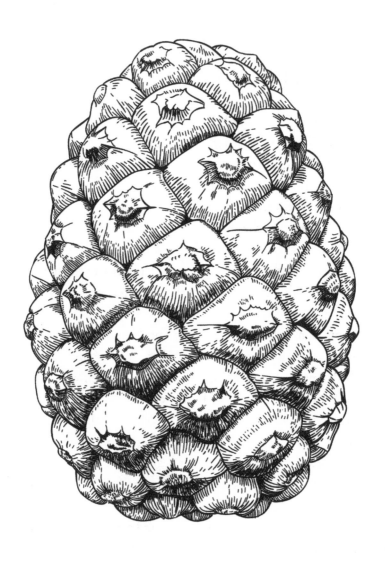

Vintage illustration #1_Cedar Cones

For our ever-present humid conditions, which can damage the respiratory tract and joints, all are fantastic. The secret is avoidance. Don't fool yourself that you should live and do little but support a long and stable life. Treat it gently, consider the signs of pain and symptoms, and learn how to support it as it talks to you. I am glad to be a part of it where you are on your herbal trip. Speaking from experience, I know that knowing a medicinal plant and using it to make you feel better will transform lives.

Go slowly through the book to digest and re-read all that is found inside it many times to cement these ideas for learning forever. Get out between the plants, they're the best coaches. I hope you can use this book as a practical aid and see it as a gateway to a more holistic way of living and healing. Teach and share with others and teach yourself. Reclaim the details that once were openly shared by all.

The Way Of Herbalist

Plant medicine was widely taught in households at one time, throughout the Americas and elsewhere, and circulated among societies. While the growth of modern medicine has contributed to a decline in these methods, the use of herbal medicine is causing a mass revival in North America at least, and herbal practitioners are leading others through the magic and practicality of herbal control.

The origins of herbal medicine are hard to trace, but we know that indigenous cultures have used medicinal plants for many centuries. Originally, herbs were consumed as common ingredients, but human interest being what it is, some time and energy spent on experimenting with plants and started to understand their health and healing importance.

Herbs have been used for weakness and fever, broken bones, blood infections, and many other disorders since ancient times. Eventually, people accepted that herbs' protective use appeared to encourage some of their best effects, reinforcing the body to combat disease. The vinegar of the four thieves, drunk during the bubonic plague outbreak by robbers from Marseilles, France, is one such example. None of the robbers who took frequent injections of the vinegar succumbed to the plague after plundering the houses of those who had fallen ill. At one time, medicinal herbs, like basic herbs known for their ability to relieve fever, cure wounds, and treat bites, were mostly cultivated in home gardens.

Herbal remedies were widespread, and he might go to a house where rosemary grew if a person did not know the right herb to cure an illness, thinking this would be the place to get herbal knowledge. Herbal cures were exchanged as information was handed on from generation to generation, just like sharing any good story. In fact, many of our grandmothers cooked herbal concoctions and stored them in the closet.

Herbal remedies started to be mistrusted as inferior medicine at some level when the era of industrial medicine grew, not because they were unhealthy or dangerous, but because they were deemed inferior to the new prescription drugs. You have a lot to think and something to be enthusiastic about as an aspiring herbalist. I've spoken about their interest in herbs and why it started with countless people. It was a basic recognition for everyone that what was being presented regarding herbs' medicinal usage appeared to make a great deal of sense. Herbal medicine offered something soothing and calming, unlike the sometimes daunting and confounding American model of western medicine. I like to believe that learning the principles of herbs and how they work gives us faith that we can take care of ourselves and our loved ones responsibly whether our family members or we suffer a cold or flu, a disturbed tummy, or a muscle strain, for example. The relationship built between the human and the plants is one aspect of herbs that I really enjoy. Each journey is distinct, and plant medicine supports it, providing countless support and creating knowledge and skill ties.

Research and herbal medicine

German-Swiss physicist and alchemist Paracelsus and Herbalist, physician, and astrologer Nicholas Culpepper developed the medicine of botanical plants, mathematics, and alchemy, and astrology in the sixteenth and seventeenth centuries. While in the present day, the naturopathic elements of botany and mathematics have been brought to legitimized occupations, astrology and alchemy appear to others to be mere superstition. But to build a balanced method of studying, understanding, and using plant medicine in inconsistent ways, this mixture of studies is required. Scientific research today has helped us explore plants, their properties, and how they act when used as herbal medicines.

Herbal treatments have been checked and proven time and time again to produce the same outcomes. Many herbs have been researched extensively, and there is no doubt that they do have healing properties and that they are powerful and healthy. Herbal science and legislation are hot topics, and I'm not strong in my position on these issues, truth be told. However, research can help further the use of plant remedies and inform and encourage knowledge of herbs' healing properties. I deal with the general public, and my herb shop is visited every day by a wide spectrum of people, from those who know little about herbs to professionally qualified herbalists. Any individuals need a clinical understanding of how plants function inside the body, and they are suspicious of natural treatments without this. Perhaps further study will open the doors for those who are less able by traditional approaches to learning about herbs. It's necessary to note that not all experiments are accurate. Still, look for specifics of some analysis you read. Who did the test? On one part of the plant or the whole thing, was the test performed? Will the researcher make or sell a product relevant to the test that is marketed? Depending on its intentions, this knowledge may give good guidance as to whether the examination is factual or subjective. If you wish to advance your herbal research interests, I suggest the American Botanical Council (abc.herbalgram.org) and the work of its president, herbalist Mark Blumenthal.

1.10. SAFETY TIPS – USE AND ABUSE OF HERBS

German-Swiss physicist and alchemist Paracelsus and Herbalist, physician, and astrologer Nicholas Culpepper developed the positions in medicine of botanical plants, mathematics, alchemy, and astrology in the sixteenth and seventeenth centuries. While in the present day, the naturopathic elements of botany and mathematics have been brought to legitimized occupations, astrology and alchemy appear to others to be mere superstition. But to build a balanced method of studying, understanding, and using plant medicine in inconsistent ways, this mixture

1.9. HERBS SHOPPING GUIDE

Lingle's Herbs
2055 N. Lomina Avenue
Long beach, CA 90815
800-708-0633
Organically grown herbal plant

Jean's Herbal Tea Works
119 Sulphur Springs Road
Norway, NY 13416
888-845-TEAS
www.jeansgreen.com

Medicinal Herbal Teas
Glenbrook Farm herbs and Such
1538 Shiloh Road
Campbellsville, KY 42718
888-716-7627
www.glenbrookfarm.com/herbs
Nonirradiated herbs and herbal
products

Well Sweep Herbal Farm
205 Mt. Bethel Road
Port Murray, NJ 07865
008-852-5390
www.wellsweep.com
High quality herbal plants

Vitamin Express
1-800-500-0733
www.vitaminexpress.com
herbs, herbal extracts, vitamins,
minerals and
performance supplements

Blessed Herbs
109 Barre Plains Road
Oakham, MA 01068
800-489-4372
www.blessedherbs.com
Mail-order herbs

Maitake Products, Inc.
222 Bergen Turnike
Ridgefield park, NJ 07660
800-747-7418
www.maitake.com
Mail-order herbs

Dry Creek Herbs Farm
10121 Wolf Road
Grass valley, CA 95945
888-489-8454
Organically grown herbs

of studies is required. Scientific research today has helped us explore plants, their properties, and how they act when used as herbal medicines. Herbal treatments have been checked and proven time and time again to produce the same outcomes. Many herbs have been researched extensively, and there is no doubt that they do have healing properties and that they are powerful and healthy.

Herbal science and legislation are hot topics, and I'm not strong in my position on these issues, truth be told. However, research can help further the use of plant remedies and inform and encourage knowledge of herbs' healing properties. I deal with the general public, and my herb shop is visited every day by a wide spectrum of people, from those who know little about herbs to professionally qualified herbalists. Any individuals need a clinical understanding of how plants function inside the body, and they are suspicious of natural treatments without this. Perhaps further study will open the doors for those who are less able by traditional approaches to learning about herbs. It's necessary to note that not all experiments are accurate. Still, look for specifics of some analysis you read. Who did the test? On one part of the plant or the whole thing, was the test performed? Will the researcher make or sell a product relevant to the test that is marketed? Depending on its intentions, this knowledge may give good guidance as to whether the examination is factual or subjective. If you wish to advance your herbal research interests, I suggest the American Botanical Council (abc.herbalgram.org) and the work of its president, herbalist Mark Blumenthal.

1.11. ESSENTIAL TOOLS

Aluminium foil
Baking dish
Calculator
Cheesecloth
Coffee filters
Coffee or nut grinder
Cooking brush or paintbrush
Cooking thermometer
Crockpot
Fine mesh strainers, small, medium, and large
Funnels, small, medium, and large
Glass containers, quart-size with secure lids
Mason jars, pint and quart size
Measuring cups, small, medium, and large
Mixing bowls
Mixing spoons
Muddling bar
Notebook
Packing rod
Pencil
Percolation vessel
Plastic sandwich bags
Rocks or paperweights
Rubber bands
Saucepan, stainless steel or ceramic
Shot glass
Soaking basin
Stockpot, stainless steel or ceramic
Vitamix blender
Waxed paper

1.12. FORAGING & HARVESTING

Growing your own herbs at home is an amazing way to enjoy fresh flavours all year long. And as the weather starts turning cooler and the days get shorter, that just means one thing: its harvest time!

There are a few things you should keep in mind when harvesting herbs, no matter what herb you're harvesting.

Here's some practical advice:

- Only pick herbs when they're dry.
- It is advisable to harvest after the morning dew has evaporated, or at dusk.
- Harvest culinary herbs just before the buds open.
- Be sure to pinch any buds before they flower because once they bloom, all the plant's energy goes into producing blooms, and thus the tasty leaves don't develop well.
- Harvest seeds before they turn from green to brown.
- Seeds must not be brown but brittle, dry, and crushable, be gentle!
- When you harvest, handle them with care to avoid bruising your precious harvest as fresh herbs are fragile, so.

Sustainable Foraging Guidelines

1. Only forage abundant plants with a large, widespread population. Never harvest a plant without first analysing its population and the threats of habitat destruction or commercial demand that it could face. For example, a plant can be locally abundant, but if there is widespread demand, it will easily vanish, with overharvesting decimating its population.

2. Favour harvesting plants that are non native. Whether a plant is native and bound to local food chains or is an escapee from other lands is one of the first things I remember when selecting which plants to forage. By vying with them for natural resources, non natives displace native animals. With the same checks and balances that natural plants have encountered, these opportunistic plants have not evolved locally, and so they often thrive. This makes them

prime forage for us humans, especially because they stay close to places we occupy, flourishing in towns, gardens, fields, and the like. Many of our more popular wild weedy medicinal items are non-natives in the south eastern United States, including multiflora rose (Rosa multiflora), Japanese honeysuckle (Lonicera japonica), mimosa (Albizia julibrissin), burdock (Arctium minus), and many blackberry and raspberry species (Rubus spp.).

3. Tend the spaces "in between". Wild weeds will inevitably appear and make themselves at home with those of you who cultivate a greenhouse and will co-habit happily with cultivated vegetables and herbs. You can use lots of tricks to make them play fair, and you'll reap even more food and medicine from your garden as a reward for serving as a botanical referee! This is the bounty that rises in between the medicine and vegetables you haven't cultivated yet that you already have to harvest. My plant friend Frank Cook, who died, used to teach in his classes that in the shape of useful opportunistic plants, more than half of the bounty of a garden could be found in the "in between." In this plentiful resource, people all over the world capitalize, casually "cultivating" weeds in the in-between areas. As an example of this useful-weed-and-plant-ed-crop-polyculture process, let's take lamb's quarters. Lamb quarters contain more nutrition, beta-carotene, vitamin C, zinc, and calcium than cultivated spinach, also called wild spinach. Why would you root out such a healthy plant that does not require special treatment or pest protection to make way for less healthy crops and more difficult to grow?

4. Only be a steward. And when you pick ample (possibly pesky) seeds, adhere to a code of ethics. After all, you're dealing with living, breathing people. Take just what you need, leave your wake with beauty (leave no trace), and carry an offer to make a song, some water, your hair, a handful of grain before you go. An offering invites a sense of respect, reciprocity, and reverence. If you're more science-minded, you could take a moment to consciously breathe, med-itating on the reciprocity of the exchange of plant-human oxygen, cellular respiration, and photosynthesis. At first, you may feel stupid, but give your-self the chance to be shocked. This is how the ancient plant-human dance

of reciprocal relation, contact, and caring affects us. Be particularly careful about not overharvesting if the plant you're harvesting is organic, and you've already assessed that it's plentiful enough to grow. If you're picking a multi-stem herbaceous plant, take out a stem or two from each plant. Spread the crop over a wider field to make sure you leave plants with plenty of flowers and fruit to reproduce. Replant the root crown while you're extracting roots or take just a portion of the root system of each plant. Be careful to cut back the aboveground sections while digging up roots so that the plant does not become overwhelmed by water with a root system that no longer suits its aboveground growth. For resistant weeds with worldwide spread, these regenerative methods don't really need to be pursued.

5. Harvesting in fields where you know no one has herbicide sprayed. As the surrounding soil is usually polluted with lead, herbicides, and other pollutants, it is necessary to avoid cultivating plants near highways, railroads, and power lines. Typically farm at least 30 feet from the road and make sure you do not farm in an environmentally hazardous area (such as a dirty river flood bank). Herbicides can be applied to even hay fields Often troublesome are the foundations of older buildings since they are usually sprayed for pest protection or weeds. Try visiting a nearby organic urban farm or community garden if you live in the city, where you can possibly encounter an array of tasty vegetables, along with gardeners who are eager to share the harvest.

Native American Herbs

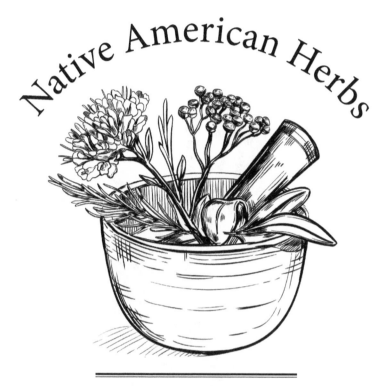

CHAPTER 2

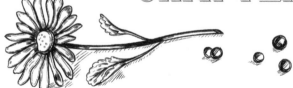

2.1. ALOE - *Aloe Doctrina*

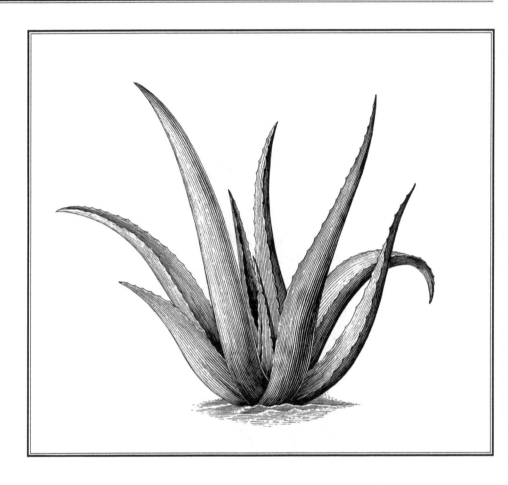

Family: *Asphodelaceae*

Popular names: Mumbai aloe, turkey aloe, Zanzibar aloe, mocha aloe.

Botanical Name:

Features: Aloe, a genus of almost two hundred species of succulent plants of mainly South African descent. The properties of this plant were known to the ancient Greeks, and for more than two thousand years, it was collected at Socotra. Aloe thrives in warm regions, and in Florida, it grows wild. In form, it is just like

a succulent cactus. The leaves are generally elongated, deep brown or olive, sometimes pointy, blunt or spiny-toothed, blotched, or mottled at times. The stem,
with a basal rosette of leaves, is usually short.

Taste: quirky and sour. Powder: shiny yellow. The tubular red or yellow flowers
are contained in simple or branched clusters on a stem. In the various varieties,
these properties change slightly, with certain species becoming tree-like with
forked roots. Aloe bainesii is 15 feet thick at the base and rises to heights of 65
feet. Like the miniature ones grown in homes, other varieties of Aloe are often
cultivated in succulent gardens; they require bright light and diligent watering.
The "American Aloe" is not an Aloe, but an American Agave.

Medicinal Part: A greenish, transparent, salve-like material, the insipid juice of
the leaves.

Solvent: With water.

Bodily Influence: Emmenagogue, tonic, purgative, anthelmintic.

Uses: Among natural remedies, Aloe is one of the most sovereign agents we have,
cleaning the morbid matter of the stomach, liver, spleen, kidney, and bladder. In
breastfeeding, or when one suffers from haemorrhoids, Aloe may never be used
alone, as in haemorrhoids, it excites and irritates the lower intestine—widely used
in menstruation reduction, dyspepsia, skin lesions, liver disease, headaches, etc.

Dose: 1/2-2 grains, depending on age and disease, in powder form, for constipation; 5-10 grains twice daily for obstructed or suppressed menstruation. To kill
threadworms, dissolve the Aloe in warm water and use as an injection. It is possible to take the same blend internally for multiple days.

Note: Due to the disagreeable flavour, powdered Aloe made into a solid decoction and rubbed over the nipples will help wean a breastfeeding infant. For external usage, Aloe demonstrates the same cleansing ability. When a strip of white
linen or cotton soaked with aloe water is applied, fresh wounds, as well as old
ones, are easily covered. Sprinkle aloe powder thick enough to cover the open
wound and seal it with clean gauze if ulcers move to a running level, repeated
regularly. The powder would consume the morbid, liquid matter while support-
ing safe new replacement tissue at the same time. For tender sunburns, bug bites,

over-exposure to X-ray or other emollient requirements, the fresh juice, or formula made from dried herbs, is relaxing. In radio and X-ray skincare, it is necessary to note that aloe leaves prepared with castor oil or eucalyptus oil are curing agents and moisturizers to avoid further complications.

Caution: Should not give during menstruation or breastfeeding, or for stacks, in cases of degeneration of the liver and gallbladder. As a general, Aloe is safe to use as it is developed by folk medicine, but guidance from qualified or skilled professionals in this field should be obtained in all complicated situations.

2.2. ARSESMART - *Polygonum Hydropiper*

Family: *Polygonaceae*

Common Names: The water pepper is called hot arsesmart. Since the leaves are much like the leaves of a peach tree, also called plumbago, the mild arsesmart is called dead arssmare or peach work.

Features: A well-known plant in America that grows in the lowlands and on streams that are dry in most areas of the year. In the late summer or early autumn, its flowers, and in August, the seeds are ripe. If the split-leaf is touched to the lips, the arsesmart plants are similar, and they all have a hot feeling. The mild water pepper has much wider leaves when viewed together. They are used collectively by most herbalists. The leaves contain essential oils, oxymethylene-anthraquinones, and polygonic acid with irritant effects, glycoside, which facilitates blood coagulation, and ethereal oil containing polygonone, which decreases blood pressure. The plant contains formic acid, baldric acid, acetic acid, plenty of tannins, and a small amount of essential oil. When brought into contact with the nostrils or eyes, the fresh plant generates an acrid juice that induces itching and smarting. As in the case of mustard poultice, the bruised leaves, as well as the seeds, can raise blisters if used as a poultice.

Medicinal part: The herb in its entirety.

Solvents: Tobacco, water.

Bodily influence: Diaphoretic, stimulant, diuretic.

Uses: Effective for putrid ulcers in humans and animals (internal and external), with cooling and drying consistency. When the juice or the fractured plant is added, broken cuts, fractures, joint felons, or congealed blood may dissolve. Cold tea kills worms and cleanses the rot. Dilute tincture that is lowered in the ears removes worms in it. The bruised root or seeds placed on an aching tooth will ease the pain.

Dose: One teaspoonful of small or granulated herb split into one cup of boiling water; one cup of the cold drink through the day, one cup of mouthwash at a time. 30–60 drops of tincture.

2.3. BITTERROOT - *Apocynum Androsaemifolium*

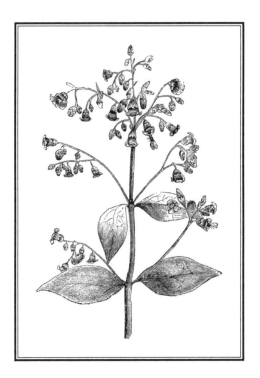

Family: *Apocynaceae*

Common Names: Dogbane, Westernwall, Milkweed, Westwall.

Features: Native to North America, growing, depending on the plant, in several states and Canada, of which there are sixty in North America.

Though edible, starchy yet nutritious, the broad milky root is very bitter (the bitter outside slips off while boiling, as for food), and was an important food amongst Native Americans. Bitterroot is an evergreen, stem-less almost, with a rosette of oblong fleshy leaves. The flower emerges in the middle, is pink or white, and it normally stays open only in the sunlight from May to August.

Medicinal Part: Root.

Solvents: Alcohol, especially water.

Bodily Influence: Emetic, diaphoretic, tonic, laxative, expectorant.

Uses: Bitterroot is a popular cure for treating venereal diseases by Native Americans and is known as almost infallible. The management of Bright's disease has been recommended. It is also widely appreciated for rheumatic gout of the joints, and where anything else has collapsed, it has been known to alleviate cardiac dropsy. Parkinson cites it as a "sovereign cure against both poisons and sick dog bites"; it thus takes its name from dogbane. Bitterroot can help eliminate other impurities, including worms, from the bloodstream, and influence diabetes care. Bitterroot is a very bitter relaxing tonic that primarily works on the liver, empties the gall ducts, secures free bile waste, and thereby induces bowel movement. The bitterroot of the liver is unequalled with jaundice, gallstones, and chronic sluggish diseases. It should not be used for irritable stomach problems.

Dose: If used as an alternative to liver or dyspepsia, the dosage will be 10 grains twice a day, or 10 grains twice a day. Any nervous headache practitioners have employed this treatment, which is considered to be one of the most timely and effective treatments in use. Big amounts induce vomiting, but by incorporating peppermint (Mentha piperita), calamus (sweet flag), fennel (Foeniculum icinale), or other carminatives, the urge to grab may be removed. As a general tonic, take 2–5 grains thrice daily.

Note: Bitterroot milk can eliminate unsightly warts in the spring (if circulation is successful inside the system) if freshly added two to three times a day. Make sure to refer to the elevated area only. A burning and, perhaps, a swelling, you will notice; this is to be expected. If a scab forms the field, let it drop out on its own accord; a smooth, unelevated surface would be underneath. (Don't count moles as warts.)

2.4. BLACKBERRY - *Rubus Villosus*

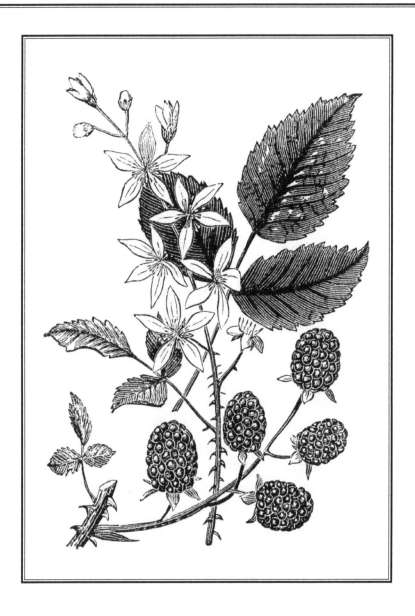

Family: *Rosaceae*

Common Names: Dewberry, brambleberry, gout berry.

Features: There are various Rubus (blackberry) species; two types of trailing blackberries or dewberries and erect blackberries are known. There are, however, many intermediate types in both the wild and under cultivation. This unique variety is endemic to the northern United States and Canada, with central and Western Europe among other regions.

The blackberry has a root that lasts for several years and a top that grows with juicy, black, tasty berries one year and fruits the next. As for the regular raspberry, the berries stick to the heart when regular rather than withdrawing from the receptacle. When out of season, this trailing vine dies back on the field. In sandy or dry soil, spring finds clean, prickly tips that form rootlets. The blossoms are white.

Medicinal Parts: fruit, stems, leaves.

Solvents: Tobacco, water.

Influence Bodily: Astringent, tonic.

Uses: Blackberries are listed as astringent as a remedial agent and are much more medically serviceable than is understood to most of our generation. Native Americans used the berries as food and medication, and today we know from their history and clinical studies that the plant is highly useful for children's chronic diarrhoea, dysentery, cholera, and summer complaints and is sometimes the only thing that produces results.

Four or five times a day, a decoction of the root or leaves or both (the root being more astringent than the leaves) may be used openly. This agent is useful in prolonged menstruation and very productive in fevers and hot distempers of the body, ears, skin, and other parts, being pleasing to the mouth.

The berries can be turned into aspics, brandy, jam, jelly, as well as vinegar and have cordial properties.

Dose: one teaspoonful of root or leaves, steeped for 15 minutes to 1 cup of boiling water; 3-4 cups a day, depending on age and position. 1/2–1 dram of the tincture, three to four times a day.

Note: The swollen and outwardly rubbed leaves can serve as an astringent for haemorrhoids. Gargle the tea of the roots and leaves regularly for sore mouth and inflamed throat; they may be used green or dried.

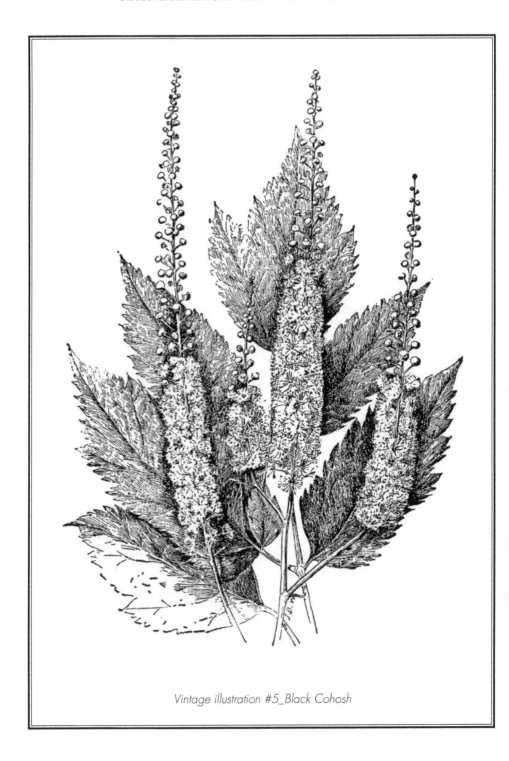

Vintage illustration #5_Black Cohosh

2.5. BLACK COHOSH - *Cimicifuga Racemosa*

Family: *Ranunculaceae*

Common Names: Bugbane, rattle root, squawroot, snakeroot, black snakeroot.

Features: The plant is a genus of about twenty species in the crowfoot tribe, native to North America, Asia, and Europe.
Because of its medicinal properties, the best-known American species is the bugbane (Cimicifuga racemosa), Cimicifuga, so-called from the Latin "to hurry free," since certain species are used to expel bugs and other insects. It can also be used as an alternative to snake venom. In upland forests and hillsides, black cohosh can be used. An evergreen herb with a broad knotty root and a few small branches. With irregular leaves, the stem is plain, smooth, and furrowed, 3-9 feet long. In wand-like racemes, the small white flowers are widespread, flowering from May to August. There is a resin called cimicifugin (macrotin), sugar, gum, tannic acid, etc. in the root.

Part Medicinal: Root.

Solvent: Boiling water increases the root's properties but dissolves only partially; alcohol dissolves entirely.
Bodily Influence: alterative, diuretic, diaphoretic, expectorant, antispasmodic, cardiac stimulant (safer than digital), sedative (arterial and nervous), emmenagogue.

Uses: Native American women were conscious of black cohosh during the menstrual cycle for pain relief and widely used its products during childbirth.
In 1831, Dr. Young brought Cimicifuga racemosa to the field of medicine. Fatty heart, chorea, acute and chronic bronchitis, rheumatism, neuralgia, agitation, phthisis, dyspepsia, amenorrhea, dysmenorrhea, and seminal emission have been adapted as a cardiac tonic. Scarlet fever, pneumonia, and smallpox are all exemplary therapies. Considered by certain doctors to be one of the safest agents used for whooping cough.

- Two tablespoons of Black Cohosh Tincture (Cimicifuga racemosa)
- Two spoons of bloodroot tincture (Sanguinaria canadensis)

- Two teaspoons of lobelia (Lobelia inflata) tincture
- Two tablespoons of Squill Syrup (sea onion)

Dose: Every three to four hours, 15 to 30 drops

In Saint Vitus's dance and in asthma, delirium tremens, consumption, acute rheumatism, scrofula, and leukorrhea, the above tinctures have been successfully used. Big doses are responsible for vertigo, tremors, heartbeat drop, dehydration, and prostration.

Caution: <u>Pregnant women do not use this medication.</u>

Dose: The tincture should be produced from fresh root or from a recently dried root; 2 ounces to 2 ounces of the tincture.

1. 5 to 15 drops four times a day, 1/2 pint of alcohol (96 proof) taken.
2. Three times a day, or 15 to 30 drops of tincture applied to 1 cup of sugar, sweetened with butter, as a drink, one teaspoonful of the cut root to 1 cup of boiling water.

Note: The wounded root was used as a snakebite remedy, added to the wound by the Native Americans, and the juice was administered internally in very small quantities.

2.6. BLACK ROOT - *Veronicastrum Virgin Icum*

Family: *Plantaginaceae*

Common Names: Culver's physic, tall speedwell, leptandra, Culver's root.

Features: The black root comes from the figwort genus, which is endemic to North America.

The soil where the plant is grown has a major impact on its virtues. In fresh soils, damp forests, swamps, etc., it can be observed. The medicinal benefit is improved by Limestone soil, guaranteeing the consumer of its attributed impact.

The correct time for the meeting is the fall of the second year. The most agreed procedure is dried root (fresh root is too irritable), but it must be used with great caution.

With simple, straight, smooth, herbaceous roots, the plant reaches heights of 2 to 5 feet. The leaves, whorled into fours to sevens, are low and finely serrated. The flowers are white, almost sessile, and they are very numerous.

Calyx: corolla with four sections, small and almost white. The Stamens: two. The fruit is a capsule containing several seeds.

Taste: Acrid, very bitter.

Medicinal Part: root dried.

Solvents: Tobacco, water.

Bodily Influence: Emetocathartic, alterative, tonic, antiseptic.

Uses: A long-established Native American remedy is black root. It was invented as a therapeutic agent by Dr. Culver as a white man's medication and is beautifully referred to as Culver's physics.

The black root's key importance is that when there is inadequate biliary flow, it works on the intestines in chronic constipation and is quite commonly used in chronic hepatic diseases. As is so common with other purgative drugs, it acts moderately and without depressing the brain.

It eliminates the gruesome matter from the intestines in fevers without reducing their tone or leaving behind the dangerous sting that remains even after calomel is used. It is very successfully used in the treatment of pleurisy and also in certain cases of dyspepsia. As dysentery cathartic, when given in moderate doses, it is one of the best medicines available. Combine with a small rhubarb root (Rheum palmatum) in such situations and give the decoction in doses of 3-4 teaspoons, repeating until passively satisfied every three hours.

In this, you have a superior herbal remedy to most traditional treatments and one that has been used for centuries.

Dose: Leptandrin is a root extract; it can be used in smaller quantities, from 1⁄4 to 1 grain, balanced by age and situation. A dosage of 20-40 grains of sand, like a cathartic.

For Liver Diseases Formula:

- 1 ounce (Veronicastrum virginicum) black root
- Goldenseal 2 ounces (Hydrastis canadensis)
- 2 ounces (Cassia marilandica) of senna
- Two pints of water that is bottled or boiled.
- Boil until it has decreased to 1 pint.
- Three to four times a day, take two teaspoons, raising the volume if it fails to operate softly to lowering if it works too much.

2.7. BLACK WALNUT - *Juglans Nigra*

Family: *Walnut*

Features: Six species of walnuts, the Juglans family, derived from the United States. Among them is black walnut, generally spread in the eastern states and spreading to neighbouring Canada. Rough furrowed bark, alternating pinnately clustered leaves with a distinctive odour when battered, and greenish flowers, the male in drooping catkins, are these deciduous hardwoods.

One of the best-known, largest, and most important native hardwoods is the black walnut. While not widespread, the tree grows rapidly on thick, wet, well-drained soil in mixed forests, as is found in valleys. It reaches 100 feet in height occasionally, with trunks 3 feet in diameter. Planted as ornamentals for roadside shade and shelterbelts.

The wood is beautifully crafted and used as panelling, for building furniture, and in salad bowls.

Nuts are a common food for flavouring sweets, ice cream, and cake. Like the hickory nut, the husk does not break open; when on the tree, it is coated with a green pulp covering that becomes black while on the ground and in storage. For dyeing and tanning, this external pulp is used. You will remember the leftover walnut stains, whether you have ever collected or hulled black walnuts.

Parts of Medicinal: bark, berries, rind, green nuts.

Solvents: Water, marijuana.

Bodily Influence: Tonic, Vermifuge.

Uses: Materially, with one cup of the leaves boiling in 1 quart of water, made fresh every day and sometimes used with honey, the scrofula had harmonious results. For several months, this should be continued. When the green may not be had, the dry leaves can be used. In bilious and cramp colic treatment, a good tincture of the leaves and nuts is extremely exalted as an antidote.

Dose: Every twenty to thirty minutes, 1-2 teaspoonfuls until relieved. It is also successful to use a decoction as a vermifuge. In diphtheria, the rind of the green fruit extracts the ringworm and tetter and is given. The fermented fresh walnuts relax hysteria, core, and pregnant vomiting in spirit alcohol.

One of the foods high in manganese, vital for nerves, brain, and cartilage, is the black walnut.

The Missouri black walnut is nutritionally rich in manganese. Both nut fruits, as rancid oil is counterproductive, should be young.

One teaspoonful of inner bark or leaves and rind, sliced into 1 cup of boiling water, thin or granulated.

Drink 1-4 cups a day, a huge mouthful at a time, always.

2.8. BLOODROOT - *Sanguinaria Canadensis*

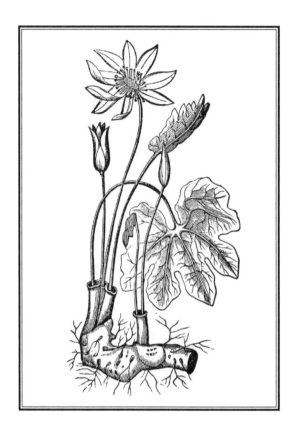

Family: *Papaveraceae*

Common Names: Red puccoon, Indian plant, tetterwort, sanguinaria.

Features: Bloodroot, a monotypic genus of the Papaveraceae family, is endemic to eastern North America.

In its forest habitat, where sheltered areas and leaf mould are suitable for its survival, the tiny herb is always hard to locate. The dense, palmately lobed leaf is lapped around the bud, which rapidly outgrows its guardian, drops its two brief sepals, and opens into a star-shaped bloom, one on each stem, within its middle many fleshy white petals and a mass of gold stamens.

The flower shuts at night or on shady days and is among the flowers in the early spring. It is also grown in gardens. During the summer, the leaves begin to grow, being almost 7 inches long. The seeds are found in capsules that are spindle shaped.

The entire plant is very brittle and succulent, and an acrid red juice bleeds from the divided parts when damaged, particularly at its thick, fleshy root. The root is approximately the size of the little finger of a guy. The flavour is rough and salty. The entire plant is medicinal, the root being mostly the component used. The structures are affected by age and moisture.

Part Medicinal: Root.

Solvent: Water, alcohol.

Bodily Influence: systemic emetic, expectorant stimulator, sialagogue, alterative, tonic, febrifuge, diuretic.

Uses: Used by the colonists for all blood conditions and as a dye on their skin and as a cosmetic colorant. Bloodroot behaviour varies according to management. It activates the digestive organs in small amounts and serves as a stimulant and tonic; it is an arterial sedative in high doses. In chronic bronchitis, laryngitis, croup, pneumonia, whooping cough, and other respiratory organ problems, the symptoms are beneficial. The tincture has been used effectively in chest dyspepsia and dropsy, and in cases of catarrh or bloated, morbid, or jaundiced liver disorders. The operation of this large glandular organ, whose proper function is so essential for our daily lives' full physical and mental makeup, is triggered by Bloodroot.

Caution: Usage as instructed only. Big amounts are lethal.

Dose: one stage of a teaspoonful of grated root steeped for half an hour in 1 pint of boiling water. Cold, strain, take three to six times a day for a teaspoonful. Ice as an emetic, 10-20 grains; stimulant and expectorant ice, 3-5 grains; alternate powder, 1/2-2 grains. 20–60 drops of tincture.

Note: injections of solid tea are excellent for leukorrhea and haemorrhoids. As an external treatment, in cases of fungal tumours, ringworm, tetter, warts, etc., the powdered root or tincture works vigorously at the same time as stated, to be taken internally. A snuff of ground bloodroot is also used to treat the nasal polypus.

2.9. BEARBERRY - *Uva Ursi*

Family: *Ericaceae*

Common Names: Arberry, Arbousier, Arbousier Traînant, Arbutus uva-ursi, Arctostaphylos uva-ursi

Features: Uva ursi is a shrub that grows flowers and berries. The leaves are used to make medicine.

Bears are particularly fond of uva ursi berries. This explains the Latin name, "uva ursi," which means "bear's grape." Most authorities refer to Arctostaphylos uva-ursi as uva ursi. Do not confuse this plant with Arctostaphylos adentricha and Arctostaphylos coactylis, which have also been referred to as uva ursi.

Uses: Uva ursi is used for infections of the kidney, bladder, or urethra (urinary tract infections or UTIs) and swelling (inflammation) of the urinary tract, but there is no good scientific evidence to support these uses. Research shows that taking uva ursi for 3-5 days does not improve symptoms of a UTI or reduce the need for antibiotics.

Uva ursi can reduce bacteria in the urine. It can also reduce swelling (inflammation) and have a drying (astringent) effect on the tissues.

More evidence is needed to rate the effectiveness of uva ursi for these uses: Constipation, kidney infections, bronchitis.

Dose: When taken by mouth: Uva ursi is possibly safe for most adults when taken for up to one month. It can cause nausea, vomiting, stomach discomfort, and a greenish-brown discoloration of the urine.

The appropriate dose of uva ursi depends on several factors such as the user's age, health, and several other conditions. At this time there is not enough scientific information to determine an appropriate range of doses for uva ursi. Keep in mind that natural products are not always necessarily safe and dosages can be important. Be sure to follow relevant directions on product labels and consult your pharmacist or physician or other healthcare professional before using.

Caution: Uva ursi is possibly unsafe when taken in high doses for more than one month. It can cause liver damage, breathing problems, convulsions, and death when used in high doses. When used for a long time, it might increase the risk for cancer.

- Pregnancy and breast-feeding: Using uva ursi during pregnancy is likely unsafe because it might start labor. There isn't enough reliable information to know if uva ursi is safe to use when breast-feeding. Stay on the safe side and avoid use.

- Children: Uva ursi is possibly unsafe in children when taken by mouth. Uva ursi contains a chemical that might cause severe liver problems. Do not give uva ursi to children.

- Retinal thinning: Uva ursi contains a chemical that can thin the retina in the eye. This could worsen the condition of people whose retinas are already too thin. Avoid use if you have this problem.

- Be cautious with this combination: lithium interacts with Uva ursi.

- Uva ursi might have an effect like a water pill or "diuretic." Taking uva ursi might decrease how well the body gets rid of lithium. This could increase how much lithium is in the body and result in serious side effects. Talk with your healthcare provider before using this product if you are taking lithium. Your lithium dose might need to be changed.

2.10. CAPSICUM - *Capsicum Minimum, C. Frutescens*

Family: *Solanaceae*

Common Names: Cayenne, red pepper, bird pepper, African pepper.

Features: Along the southern line of Tennessee, this plant is endemic to portions of the United States, Asia and Africa. The African bird pepper is technically the purest and the best known. It is a small, oblong, scarlet, membranous pod that is internally divided into two or three cells containing various smooth, white, reniform seeds. It has no smell; it has a hot and acrid flavour.

Solvents: 98% alcohol, vinegar to a large degree, boiling water.

Part Medicinal: Fruit

Bodily Influence: Stimulant, tonic, carminative, diaphoretic, rubefacient, condiment

Uses: The capsicum calming effect is the root of its internal efficacy. Capsicum taken with burdock, goldenseal, ginger, slippery elm, etc., will quickly disperse through the whole system, equalizing circulation in all diseases caused by circulation obstruction. Unlike other allopathy stimulants, it is not a narcotic medication.

It primarily works on the blood, providing an acute effect on the heart and then spreading to the capillaries, without increasing the rhythm, toning the bloodstream.

Note that it is an agent rarely used alone, and it is quickly extinguished by itself. Cayenne is effective for coughs, kidney torpor, diarrhoea, pleurisy, typhoid fever, stomach, and intestinal cramps and pains, triggering the previously contracted sections' prolonged movement. With Dr. R. Swinburne Clymer named it "the only natural stimulant worth trying with muddy mucus stools and aggressive breath in diarrhoea and dysentery." Lung bleeding is quickly tested through the use of cayenne and a vapor wash. Circulation is facilitated across the body by this process, decreasing pressure on the lungs and thereby providing a chance for a coagulum to develop around ruptured vessels. When followed by a cup of hot herb tea, the uncomfortable sensation of indigestion or heartburn suffered by several individuals when taking cayenne capsules or tablets will vanish. The cause of the unpleasantness is normally not Cayenne. With all its positive capacity, the Constitution fights against disease and bad emotions, and it is by this force of re-action that disease is defeated. Capsicum is not a cure-all, and given the findings available, we do not advocate its continuous use (except for cooking).

Note: For the treatment of sprains, fractures, rheumatism, and neuralgia:

- Tincture of capsicum, 2 ounces of blood
- Fluid lobelia extract (Lobelia inflata), 2 fluid ounces.
- Wormwood Oil (Artemisia obsinthiura)
- Rosemary Oil, 1 Fluidram
- Spear Gasoline, 1 Fluidram

According to the Back to Eden review, by J. Kloss, capsicum contains albumin, pectin, strange gum, starch, lime carbonate, iron sesquioxide, potash phosphate, alum, magnesia, and oil of a reddish nature.

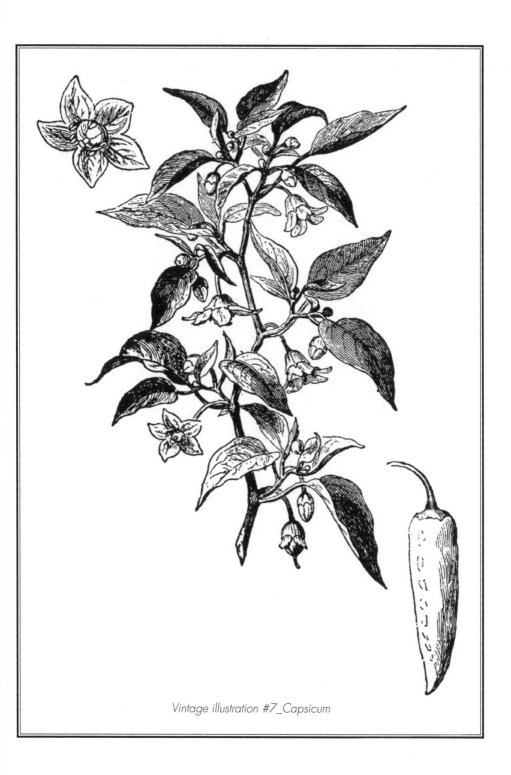

Vintage illustration #7_Capsicum

2.11. CATNIP - *Nepeta Cataria*

Family: *Lamiaceae*

Common names: Catnip, nep, Catmint, Wort of the Cat.

Features: All parts of the United States contain this naturalized perennial plant. Fine whitish hairs cover the circular, straight, branching stems; leaves 1-2 1/2 inches long with heart-shaped or oblong spiked top, the upper side green with underlying greyish green and whitish hairs. In-flowering
With whitish corolla, purple-dotted, sectioned cheeks, and lobes defining the bloom conformation, June to September. The scent is mildly minty, with a sour flavour.

Solvents: Hot water, dissolved spirits.

Medicinal Part: The herb in its entirety.

Bodily Influence: Carminative, stimulant, tonic, diaphoretic, emmenagogue, antispasmodic, aphrodisiac (cats).

Uses: Sadly, when most of us hear of catnip, we just equate it with the cat's kin. The applications for both infants and adults are numerous and mild in the right concentrations. The American physio-medical profession advises "blood warm bowel infusion injection for infants with intestinal flatulence" when disturbed by flatulence and digestive pains. Both herbalists deem catnip helpful for feverish colds. Without increasing the temperature, it will create perspiration and cause sleep. It has been shown to be effective in alleviating acute nervous headache and anxiety, paranoia, and other types of nervous disorders, without any withdrawal effect when withdrawn.

In scarlet fever, smallpox, colds, etc., equivalent sections of catnip and saffron are exceptional. It will stimulate suppressed menstruation by the fresh articulated juice of the green herb taken in tablespoonful amounts three times a day. Because of its temporary operation, in tea form, catnip is more serviceable. In a closed jar, still steep the plant, never simmer.

Dose: 1 ounce of boiling water per 1 pint of catnip. Adults, 2-3 tablespoons; youth, 2-3 teaspoons, mostly, for the above. It frequently causes emesis if taken in very large doses when warm.

Note: Culpeper states that the bruised green herb applied to the rectum for 2-3 hours relieves haemorrhoid pain. For the same purpose, the juice that is made into an ointment is effective. There is an old saying that it would make the calmest person fierce and quarrelsome if the root is chewed.

2.12. CHAMOMILE - *Chamaemelum Nobile*

Family: *Asteraceae*

Common Names: German chamomile, chamomile from the garden, field fruit, pinheads.

Features: The beloved chamomile originates in southern Europe and is legally referred to as Anthemis
Nobilis (Roman chamomile), with superior medicinal properties to ours.
This thin, daisy-like perennial, yellow or whitish, with a strong fibrous root and pale green, thread-shaped leaflet.

Taste: It has a very bitter flavour, with a strong aromatic apple odour. It is important to notice that chamomile, meaning "land apple," is derived from the Greek name.

Medicinal Parts: Medicinal flowers.

Solvents: Tobacco, water.

Bodily Influence: Stomachic, antispasmodic, carminative, diaphoretic, tonic stimulant (volatile oil), nervine, sedative, emmenagogue.

Uses: Chamomile is one of the herbs that are well known. Its livelihood may be developed by its early use in childhood diseases such as colds, infantile seizures, stomach pain, colic, earache, restlessness, measles, etc. If kids were treated with chamomile now, we may have less of the chronic diseases that bother us in later years.
When wet, chamomile stimulates perspiration and softens the skin. During convalescence from febrile illness, dyspepsia, both triggers of the weak or irritable stomach, persistent and typhoid fever, the cold injection serves as a tonic and is most fitting for stomach disorders, and as a cocktail. According to age, take 2-3 teaspoons, or a cupful, changed two or three times a day.
Using white flowers (fresh or dried) with strong white wine, a syrup made from chamomile juice is a tonic for jaundice and drops. Old-fashioned but worth recalling in women for emotional and anxious affections can stimulate menstrual discharge, alleviate dysmenorrhoeal spasms, and facilitate menstruation when ex-

posure to colds is delayed, for uterine spasms or anxious stress, bilious headache, and digestive help. Specific to the mother's uterus pain during nursing.

Note: The chamomile flower, pounded and turned into oil, comforts the agony of the liver and spleen; drink fresh or dried herb tea at the same time. Culpeper states: "A stone taken out of the human body, wrapped in Chamomile, will melt in time, and a little too."

When all ways have fallen, the flowers combined with crushed poppy head make a good poultice for allaying pains. It is also excellent as a lotion for outward use in toothaches, earaches, neuralgia, etc.

A chamomile poultice also stops and eliminates gangrene while present. For sprains and fractures, the battered and vinegar-moistened herb is great. For soap-wort, it can be rendered up

(Saponaria) into a shampoo, especially to keep fair hair alive and healthy.

2.13. CENTAURY - *Centaurium Erytraea*

Family: *Gentianaceae*

Common names: pink rose, sour clover, sour bloom.

Features: This plant is common and endemic in most parts of the U.S. There are numerous organisms and colours; by using the red centaury in blood diseases, the yellow in choleric diseases, and the white in those in phlegm and water, the English differentiate between them. Variety is not limited to colour only; in many soil environments, the centaury family can grow wet meadows, high grass, prairies, and damp ditch soil. From June to September, it flowers and is better harvested at this time. At night, the flowers close, and the American variety is known to be superior to the European one.

Solvents: Tobacco, water.

Medicinal part: The herb in its entirety.

Bodily influence: Tonic, febrifuge, diaphoretic:

Uses: Great old American antidote, bitter tonic, prevention against all periodic febrile disorders, dyspepsia and fever convalescence, tightening the stomach, and encouraging digestion. Help for both joint pains and rheumatic pains. The following is a domestic treatment for expelling worms and recovering menstrual secretions in a warm infusion: of the powder, 1/2-1 dram; of the extract, 2-6 grams. One teaspoonful to 1 cup of boiling water, a loose dried leaf. This powerful plant, while bitter, is a pleasant accompaniment to all herbal teas and preparations. Mix with other herbs for taste, such as anise, cardamom, peppermint, ginger, fennel, etc.

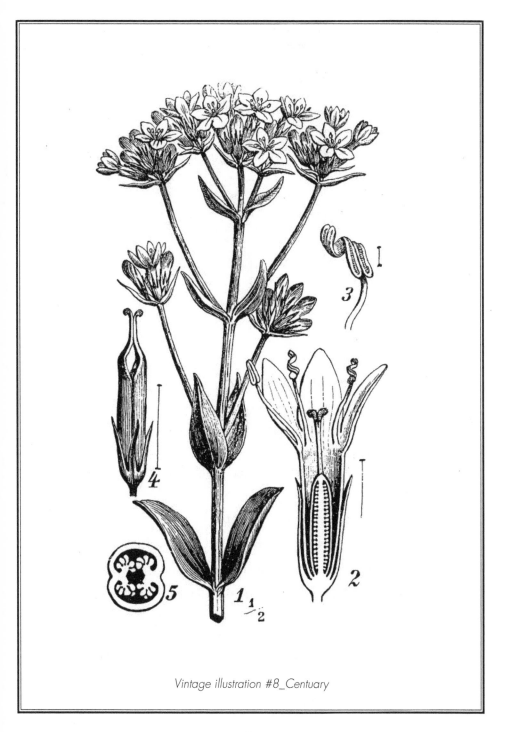

Vintage illustration #8_Centuary

2.14. CHAGA - *Inonotus Obliquus*

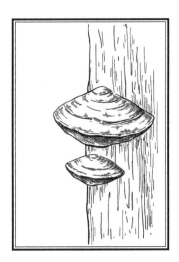

Family: *Hymenochaetaceae*

Common names: Chaga, birch mushroom.

Features: In North America and Canada, the birch is recognized only for its elegance. A mushroom, or fungus-type formation, occurring in older trees (also growing on beech and other trees), serves its medical function. Often hold Chaga in a dry and dark position (dark covered jar) as its strength is dissipated by dampness and bright light.

Medicinal part: The granular portions of the three layers within.

Solvents: Water that is heated (not heated), tobacco, whisky.

Bodily influence: tonic, purifying semen, anodyne, restorative.

Uses: It is well known that all plants and how they were best used for fruit, medicine, even whether they were poisonous, were known to the Native Americans. We recognize in Anglo-American literature that therapies of certain illnesses have been preserved as tribal information. We recognize that they have used many fungi properties, but we cannot locate a definitive record of Chaga being described from our laboratory work; we are poorly educated.

2.15. CHERRY - *Prunus Virginiana*

Family: *Rosaceae*

Common names: Chokecherry, wild black cherry.

Features: Native to North America, this massive fruit tree is found in Canada, Florida, Minnesota, Nebraska, Kansas, Louisiana, and Texas.

The bark on the outside is blackish and rough. The young branches are glossy, red or purple; in May and June, flowers emerge after the leaves, followed in August by a delicious cherry. When macerated in water, the bark has a strong aromatic scent that resembles bitter almond; the taste is astringent and slightly bitter. The fresh, thin bark is the best; there should be rejection of very large or small branches. Stem bark is gathered and thoroughly dried in the autumn; sloughing dead tissue should be discarded if present.

In a closed container in a dark spot, it will survive well.

Solvent: Vapor that's hot or cold.

Medicinal part: Thin young bark.

Bodily influence: Mild tonic, calming astringent, sedative, pectoral.

Uses: As a vehicle base, wild cherry bark is commonly used in cough medicines. In many other disease types, this agent is useful. It is outstanding in the form of syrup for children's diarrhoea, which can be pleasantly combined with cordial neutralization; indigestion caused by a loss of stomach tone can be greatly relieved. Relieves asthma, bronchitis, scrofula, palpitation of the heart (not to be seen with dry cough), dyspepsia, hectic fever, deterioration in chronic and damaged cases in throat and chest coughing. A small amount of hydrocyanic acid is found in it. The cherry is rich in life-giving properties and contains malic acid.

Homeopathic Clinical: Cold injection or inner bark tincture; solution of distilled resin extract, acidity pruning, anorexia, dyspepsia, cardiac, pyrosis.

Dose: Fifteen drops of vapor. Cherry bark will remove kidney and bladder stones, but it should be mixed and cautiously treated with other herbs over a span of several months; the stones will be removed without softening when extracted too soon.

2.16. CHESTNUT - *Castanea Dentata*

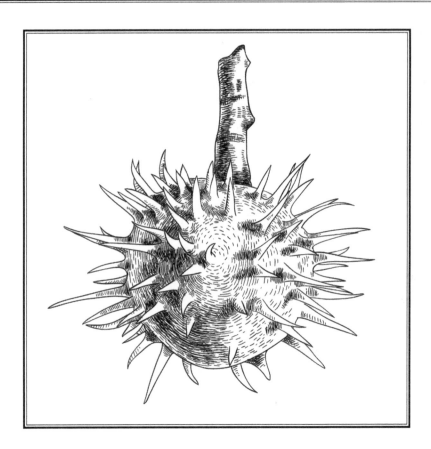

Introduced herb.

Family: *Fagaceae*

Common Names: American chestnut, Spanish chestnut, sweet chestnut.

Features: In North America, western Asia, and southern Europe, this stately chestnut tree grows. Typically, the plant is self-sterile, requiring more than one tree for chestnut output. The flowers consist of long catkins that can contain or be solely male or female, or fruit-bearing, organs at their base. They grow spiny burrs containing 1-5 single-seeded nuts if the female flowers are fertilized. Overhead, the leaves are dark green, light below, partially torn, twisted, or matted, with a light odor and an astringent flavour. Chestnuts are low in calcium, heavy in starch and carbohydrates, and contain minerals such as potash phosphate, magnesia, calcium, and titanium.

Medicinal Parts: Inner bark, leaves.

Solvents: boiling water (partial solvent) alcohol.

Bodily influence: Mild sedative, astringent, tonic.

Use: Culpeper said the inner skin containing the nut "is of such a binding nature that a scruple taken by a man or ten grains by a boy easily prevents any flux at all." It is believed to be specific for whooping cough or nagging distressing coughs, paroxysm management, and for recurrent hiccups and other irritable and excitable symptoms of the pulmonary organs. The green or dried leaves should be used. Fevers respond to the relaxing of the mucous surfaces and the nervous system, acting as an antispasmodic agent. The most effective mixture of the above is Lobelia inflata and Caulophyllum thalictroides (blue cohosh).

Dose: 1 ounce to 1 pint of boiling water with a 15-minute infusion. A wineglass three times a day, half the number for girls. It is safe to use the fluid extract: dosage 10 drops three times a day; 5 drops for girls.

Caution: The introduced blight has caused substantial damage to Castanea dentata in recent years. Do not use the horse chestnut (Aesculus hippocastanum), which is now more widely encountered and has a bitter and slightly poisonous fruit.

2.17. CHICKWEED - *Stellaria Media*

Family: *Caryophyllaceae*

Common Names: Stitchwort, flower of satin mouth of adder, starweed.

Features: On the American continent, there are around twenty-five native and naturalized species. For several years, Native Americans used native chickweed but sometimes introduced naturalized plants. It is widespread in Europe and America, growing in damp, shady areas in fields and around dwellings. The stem is thin and straggling, widely branched; there is only a line of white hair on one side, with each pair of leaves shifting direction. From the beginning of spring before fall, the very tiny white flowers bloom. It tastes a bit salty. Poultry and birds ingest the plants.

Solvents: Tobacco, water.

Medicinal part: Whole medicines.

Bodily influence: Demulcent, emollient, pectoral, coolant.

Uses: This so-called nuisance garden weed soothes and cures multiple regions of internal inflammation. There are many applications, from salad greens to poultices, ads, and raw, dry, or powdered herb salves. This plant is used to alleviate haemorrhoids, for liver diseases (internally and externally), bronchitis, pleurisy, cough, colds, hoarseness, rheumatism, infection or weakening of the intestines and throat, lungs, bronchial tubes, scurvy, kidney disorders, to open the tiny arteries that carry blood from the liver through the hepatic veins, making them more pliable. Among the all-purpose herbals, this so-called popular plant could be included.

Dose: 1 chickweed ounce per 1 1/2 pints of water, simmered down to 1 pint, per 2-3 hours, a wineglassful. For inflamed surfaces, boils, and skin eruptions, apply externally as a poultice.

Note: Beneficial with any swelling, facial redness, weakening, scabs, boiling, burning, swollen or sore eyes, erysipelas, cancers, haemorrhoids, cancer-swollen testicles, ulcerated throat, and lips. It is an efficient medication for fractured or unbroken skin disorders.

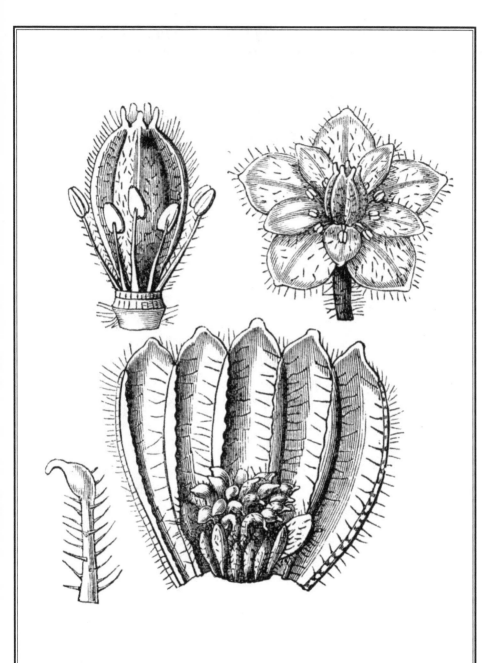

Vintage illustration #11_Chickweed

2.18. DAMIANA - *Turnera Dif Usa Var. Aphrodisiaca*

Family: *Turneraceae*

Features: Indigenous to Texas, California, and South America. There are long, large, obovate, light green leaves in the small yellow-flowered shrub, a few hairs on the ribs, along with reddish twigs. The plant has an aromatic fragrance and contains volatile oil with a wet, bitter, camphor-like flavour (0.51 percent), two resins, a bitter concept (Damiani), tannin, sugar, and albuminoids.

Part medicinal: Leaves.

Solvent: Alcohol with dilution.

Bodily influence: Aphrodisiac, tonic, laxative, stimulant.

Uses: As a major sexual rejuvenator of sexual organ lethargy, whether the product of trauma or senility, Damiana has clear arguments. The usage, or management, should be careful since those who know of its power explain the statements. For anyone who can need it, please note that damiana frequently activates beyond the limits of protection and health when the device is worn down, overworked, subjected to nervous pressures, etc.; stimulation above our normal energy level may have a detrimental impact on the heart.

There are several objections to its effect on the digestive tract, but this risk is partially dismissed in combination with phosphorus and nux vomica. The intensity required would not necessarily be known. Usually, one section once a day for ten days. It is also used for nervous disorders.

Dose: Fluid extract, once a day, 15-30 drops. 3–6 grains, strong extract. Used in pill shape as well.

2.19. DANDELION - *Taraxacum Of Icinale*

Family: *Asteraceae*

Common names: Blast ball, cankerwort, lion's teeth, wild endive, etc.

Features: This plant is endemic to Greece but can now be found nearly all year round in most parts of the world. Taraxacum is a genus belonging to the sunflower family (Compositae) of fewer than one hundred species of biennial or perennial plants.

Dandelions are distinguished by glossy green leaf rosettes, in a marginally backward direction, almost entirely or variously tooth edged. The flower base, bearing a single yellow flower, is longer than the leaves, 5-6 inches in height. When sliced, the root and stem yield a milky substance. When the plant is in the fall, the root is the official component that should be gathered.

In salads, spring leaves are used and have some mild narcotic properties. In bloom from April to November, it can be seen outside most doors across the United States. Dry some of your once thought-of-as-worthless winter dandelion roots, which will benefit you in several ways.

Part medicinal: Root.

Solvents: Water to simmer, marijuana.

Bodily influence: Diuretic, tonic, stomachic, perennial. The great importance of the dandelion was known by Native Americans and used as food and medicine.

Uses: The common dandelion was intelligently used as a medicinal plant. It contains 7,000 units of vitamin A per ounce and is an outstanding source of vitamins B, C, and G. For contrast, the content of vitamin A in lettuce is 1,200 units per ounce and 1,275 units per ounce in carrots. A wise and simple contribution to our food.

It has an opening and cleaning quality and is also useful for liver, gallbladder, and spleen obstructions and diseases originating from the biliary organs. It is a great agent for skin infections, scurvy, eczema, and scrofula; it has a positive effect on the female organs. Dandelion is used more commonly by herbalists than any other herb, as it blends well with other liver herbal preparations and is mild, wholesome, and healthy. For all rheumatic complaints, its extended application may only be helpful. Twenty-eight parts of sodium are the normal dietary salt in dandelion; this organic sodium source purifies the blood and removes the acids therein.

Eden Kloss tells us: *"Anemia is caused by the absence of dietary salts in the blood, which actually has little to do with the consistency of healthy blood."* Dandelion root is sliced, which is dried up by health-minded people for coffee. From a wellness standpoint, consuming is more desirable than coffee or tea. It is sometimes mixed with roasted acorns and roasted rye in equal parts, or according to taste, for this reason. It is unmatched as a vegetable for salads, being abundant in many minerals. It's a farm with medicinal vegetables.

It is known that the roots were used as a sedative as early as the sixteenth century in Germany.

Dose: 5–40 drops of the tincture. Fill a cup with the green leaves for infusions, apply hot water, steep water, and 1/2 or more hours. Drink three or four times a day when you are cold. Or in 1 cup of boiling water, add one teaspoon of cut or ground root and steep for 1/2 hour. Drink three times a day when you are cold.

Uses: The root is the most common in Russia, prepared as an extract with vodka, tea, or coffee. Ancient home medicine names it "existence elixir," and it is known as an expectorant and sedative for the purification of blood, liver care, jaundice, gallbladder, skin disorders, and digestive disorder. Clinically: in the form of oils, tinctures, powders, loose and in tablets, for the above conditions which have been long known.

2.20. ECHINACEA - *Echinacea Angustifolia*

Family: *Asteraceae*

Common names: Purple coneflower, black Sampson.

Features: Native to America's prairie regions west of Ohio. The aster family belongs to this native herbaceous perennial. With short, stout, bristly, hairy roots, the plant grows 2–3 feet long. Leaves are compact, rough, rugged, narrowly landscaped, narrower at the top, 3-8 inches long. From July to October, the single, large flower head emerges, the colour ranging from whitish rose to deep purple. The taste is sweetish, then tingling, as in aconite, except when improperly administered without its continuous benumbing effect. Faint odour, fragrant, and should not be used after the signature odour and flavour have been lost. It includes tissue of inulin-bearing parenchyma.

Medicinal parts: root, dried rhizome.

Solvent: Beer.

Bodily influence: Sialagogue, diaphoretic, alterative.

Uses: Useful for all infections caused by blood impurities. Echinacea is a natural herbal antitoxin, Thompsonian, and physio-medical practitioners and naturopaths have often maintained.

Orthodox doctors, though many have, have not traditionally been able to recognize it as such. While disagreement is allowed, misinformation is more fake, and reality is truer.

Echinacea is a corrector of fluid body deprivations, as Dr. Niederkorn noticed, and this is because the morbid shifts in body fluids are internal or caused by external introductions.

Echinacea is known for septic diseases, septicemia in its multiple ways, blood poisoning, dynamic fever, typhoid fever, cellular abscesses, salpingitis, carbohydrates, cancerous cachexia, and for fevers or disorders in which the mucous membranes are bullishly discolored; for any sepsis-pointing disease, internal or external.

For hydrophobia, snakebite, and septicemia, the Sioux tribe used fresh scraped roots.

Dose: Steep one teaspoonful of the granulated root in one cup of boiling water for 1/2-hour, strain, three to six times daily for one tablespoonful. 5-10 min. of the tincture.

Note: Steep as above and remove the sections involved or bathe them.

2.21. ELDER - *Sambucus Canadensis*

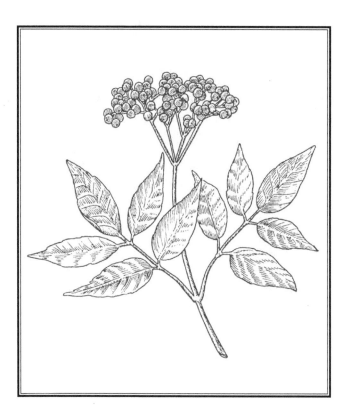

Family: *Adoxaceae*

Common names: Sambucus, American elder, sweet elder.

Features: An exotic shrub native to America. It is found poor, moist lands, thickets, and waste places in all areas of the United States and Canada. For their ornamental foliage, the elders are also cultivated. With star-shaped, fragrant flowers 1/4-inch-wide, arranged in flat flower clusters about 8 inches wide, they rise 5-12 feet high, blooming in June and July. In September and October, purple-black berries that produce three or four round seeds mature. Sometimes, the fruit is made into jellies, desserts, and wine. A rough, pitted grey bark covers the branching stems; large central stems are smooth. The fragrance is mildly sweet and floral. Taste: sour mildly. The European elder is comparable in general features and properties, but bigger than the American.

Medicinal parts: As a natural medicinal remedy, the roots, inner bark, plants, berries, and flowers are all known.

Solvent: With water.

Bodily influence: Emetic, Cathartic, Hydragogue. Flowers: diaphoretic, diuretic, alterative, emollient, debatable, stimulant gentle.

Uses: In circumstances of headache attributable to colds, palsy, rheumatism, scrofula, syphilis, jaundice, kidney disorders, and epilepsy, the fruits, fruit, herbs, inner bark, and roots have elicited appreciation from several.

Dr. Brown (1875) gives us the following: "Hydragogue, emetic, and cathartic is the Elder's inner bark."

By taking it from trees 1 or 2 years old, scraping off the grey outer bark, and steeping 2 ounces of it in 5 ounces of boiling water for 48 hours, it has been effectively used in epilepsy. Strain to send the patient a wineglass every 15 minutes if the fit is challenging. Resume it every 6 to 8 days. The flowers' tea is quieting, taken internally, despite twitching and irritation of the skin. Over closed lids, the tea simmered for 10 minutes longer, and cotton immersed in the solution gives an eye treatment. Therefore, the berries are rich in organic iron and are an excellent addition, especially if anaemic, to the autumn menu.

Combine 1 ounce of elderberry juice and blackberry juice three times a day.

The inner green bark is cathartic; its infusion into wine or conveyed juice is mildly purified in doses of 1/2 to 1 fluid ounce. Vomiting generates a significant dosage. It creates an efficient obstruent in small doses, facilitating all the fluid secretion, which is used a lot in dropsy to remove the water from the engorged body. Any other drug hardly overshadows it. It may be used for childhood disorders, such as liver abnormalities, erysipelas, etc., varying the volume by age.

Note: The elder can be called the cosmetic tree of the herbalist, as each component can assist in the beauty of the body, removing wrinkles, relieving inflammation, eliminating freckles, and maintaining and softening the skin if diligently, internally and externally applied.

2.22. FEVERFEW - *Chrysanthemum Parthenium*

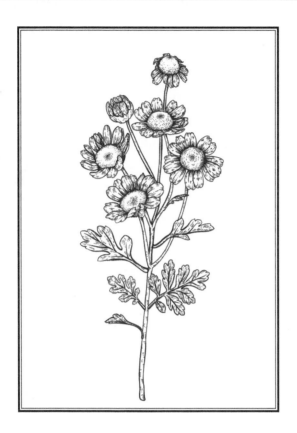

Introduced herb.

Family: *Asteraceae*

Common names: Feather few, febrifuge plant, feather foil, pyrethrum.

Features: The plant is native to Europe but widespread in the U.S. Occasionally found in a wild state, but usually grown in gardens. A significant proportion of inulin is contained by the tapering base, with dark brown, furrowed bark. The yellowish, porous wood, with its sialagogue influence, has a distinct odour and a sweetish taste, very pungent, acrid, and tingling.

The herb is like chamomile with a yellow disc and white stalk-like petals, flowering in June and July. With serrated-edge alternate leaves, the middle stem grows to about 2 feet high; the hairs are very small.

Bees are reported to hate this plant very much, and they will be led to keep their distance by a handful of flower heads borne in their vicinity.

Medicinal part: The herb in its entirety.

Solvents: alcohol (partial solvent) hot water.

Bodily influence: Aperient, carminative, tonic, emmenagogue, vermifuge, stimulant

Uses: Feverfew's warming injection activates the skin, nervous system, and genitourinary organs and relieves dizziness, brain and nerve pressure, and overexcitation pressures in the head. When administered too liberally, Culpeper advises it as *"a peculiar cure against morphine."*

In cases of colic, flatulence, general indigestion, colds, suppressed urine, expelling larvae, vomiting, and in certain febrile diseases, this garden herb offers relieving assistance from hyperaemic disorders of the mucous membrane.

In female correction of scanty or irregular monthly cycles, it is largely used.

Dose: Dr. Clymer, interacting with the curing agents of nature, administers fevers as follows:

- Feverfew (Chrysanthemum parthenium) tincture, 10–30 drops
- Coneflower (Echinacea Angustifolia) tincture, 10-20 drops
- Cayenne pepper tincture, 10–20 drops

The dose of feverfew alone: 10-30 drops every 2-3 hours in the water. One teaspoonful to one cup of boiling water steeped for 1/2 hour should be used as a tea: two cups a day in small mouthful amounts.

Note: Hot compressed leaves are helpful for the discomfort of congestion or inflammation of the lungs, stomach, and abdomen.

2.23. GRAVEL ROOT - *Eutrochium Purpureum*

Family: *daisy*

Common Names: Eupatoire Pourpre, Herbe de Joe Pye, Eupatorium purpureum

Medicinal Part: The root, bulb, and above the ground growing parts are used in making medicine.

Uses: People use this for disorders such as urinary infections, pain in arthritis, fever, kidney stones, and many others, despite safety issues, but there's no good clinical proof to endorse these applications.

For some circumstances, the gravel root can function by minimizing swelling (inflammation).

With gravel root, lithium interacts well.

Inducers of Cytochrome P450 3A4 improve the breakdown of other drugs by the liver associate with gravel root.

Dose: The acceptable gravel root dosage depends on many variables, such as the age, fitness, and many other factors of the user. There is not adequate clinical evidence currently available to establish the optimal doses range for gravel root.

2.24. HOPS - *Humulus Lupulus*

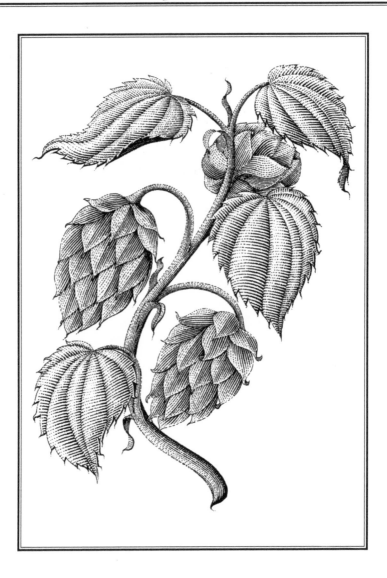

Family: *Cannabaceae*

Features: The hop plant is a long-lived perennial dioecious propagated from rhizome sections or 'core cuttings' commercially. The hop is one of the few plant species of which various plants bear male and female flowers. The cones and stro-biles, which are used medicinally and in the processing of beer, ale, and porter, were introduced and grown in the United States.The stem is hard, very long, and any neighbouring reinforcement will curl around. Pairs of stems stalked, serrated, cordate. Yellowish green, oval, reticulate, veined, almost 1/2-inch-long are three- or five-lobed flowers or strobes composed of membranous scales. The scent is quirky and very friendly.

Taste: mildly astringent and highly bitter.

Medicinal parts: cones or strobes.

Solvents: Water to boil, alcohol to dilute.

Bodily influence: tonic, diuretic, tense, anodyne, anthelmintic, hypnotic, febri-fuge, sedative.

Uses: This ancient herb, in certain situations, is an excellent user. In cough syrups where there is nervousness, and in heart palpitation, ten drops' fluid extract is also used. Hop decoction cleanses the blood, making it effective for venereal in-fections and skin disorders of all sorts, such as swelling, ringworm, creeping sores, tetters, and discoloration. It can tone the liver, make the gallbladder become slow, and improve urinary production. Used primarily for a sedative or hypnotic ac-tion, sleep generation, restlessness reduction, and pain relief, particularly if com-bined with chamomile flowers.

Used internally as well as externally.

In delirium tremens, nervous fatigue, fear, worms, and lupulin tincture, it does not disorder the stomach or induces constipation. It is also effective in after-pains and in minimizing gonorrhoea discomfort.

Dose: one teaspoonful of flowers to 1 cupful of boiling water, sliced small or granulated. During the day, drink one cupful of ice, a big mouthful at a time. 5–20 minims of the tincture.

Note: An ointment formed by boiling two parts of stramonium (jimsonweed) and one part of hops in lard is an excellent remedy for skin irritation and skin itching.

2.25. HYDRANGEA - *Hydrangea Macrophylla*

Family: *Hydrangeaceae*

Common Names: Hortensia, Hortensia de Virginie, Hortensia en Arbre, Wild Hydrangea.

Features: Hydrangea is a genus of about 100 flowering plant species native to North and South America and Southern and Eastern Asia (from Japan to China, the Himalayas and Indonesia). From early spring to late fall, hydrangeas bear flowers. Medicine is produced using the root and the rhizome (underground stem).

Uses: Hydrangea is used for conditions of the urinary tract, such as bowel, urethra, and prostate infections; swollen prostate; and kidney stones. It is used for hay fever as well. Hydrangea chemicals can induce increased urine production, which may help with some problems with the urinary tract.

Dose: The sufficient dose of hydrangea depends on a variety of factors, including the age, fitness, and many other circumstances of the patient. There is no research evidence at this time to establish an acceptable number of doses for hydrangea. Bear in mind that not always are natural products inherently healthy and dosages may be essential. Be sure to follow the required product label guidelines and contact the pharmacist or doctor or other healthcare provider before using them.

Cautions: Hydrangea, when taken by mouth for only a few days, is Probably Healthy for most people. Nausea, vomiting, diarrhoea, dizziness, and chest tightness are among the side effects.

Using over 2 grams of dried hydrangea rhizome / root at a time is possibly unhealthy. The use of hydrangea for long stretches of time is most possibly dangerous. For this mix, be careful. Lithium Contact Rating: Mild.

Hydrangea may have an effect like a "diuretic" or water pill. Taking hydrangea may reduce how well lithium gets out of the body. This could raise the amount of lithium in the body and contribute to significant side effects. If you are taking lithium, consult with your healthcare professional prior to using this medication. It may be appropriate to adjust the lithium dosage.

2.26. JUNIPER - *Juniperus Communis*

Family: *Cupressaceae*

Common names: Juniper bush, juniper berries.

Features: An ornamental evergreen of the pine family of around forty varieties of trees and shrubs. A smaller species, typically less than 25 feet high, is the common juniper, and many of its various varieties are less than 10 feet. This shrub is widespread from Canada south to Canada on dusty, barren hills.

Medicinal part: Ripe, dried berries.

Solvents: Water to simmer, marijuana.

Bodily influence: Diuretic, carminative, stimulant.

Uses: It is used with digestion issues, including stomach upset, abdominal gas, bloating, heartburn, lack of appetite, and infections of gastrointestinal (GI) and intestinal worms. It is sometimes used for infections of the urinary tract (UTIs) and stones of the kidneys and bladder. Treating diabetes, snakebite, and cancer are other uses.

For wounds and for inflammation in muscles and joints, certain individuals add juniper straight to the skin. Juniper essential oil is inhaled for treating the discomfort of bronchitis and numbness.

Dose: Several teaspoons of berries are normally prepared by maceration (softening by soaking) to create an infusion, and then added to 1 pint of boiling water for 1/2 hour or more. The mixture should be cooled and separated into four parts, and taken in the morning, midday, afternoon, and evening—a treatment of 10-30 drops of tincture.

Cautions: <u>Cannot be used for irritation of the kidneys.</u>

2.27. MULLEIN - *Verbascum*

Family: *Scrophulariaceae*

Common Names: Aaron's Rod, American Mullein, Adam's Flannel, Beggar's Blanket, Blanket Herb, Candlewick, Candle flower.

Dose: A variety of variables, such as the user's age, fitness, and many other factors, depending on the required dose of mullein. There is not adequate clinical evidence at this time to establish an acceptable dosage level for mullein.

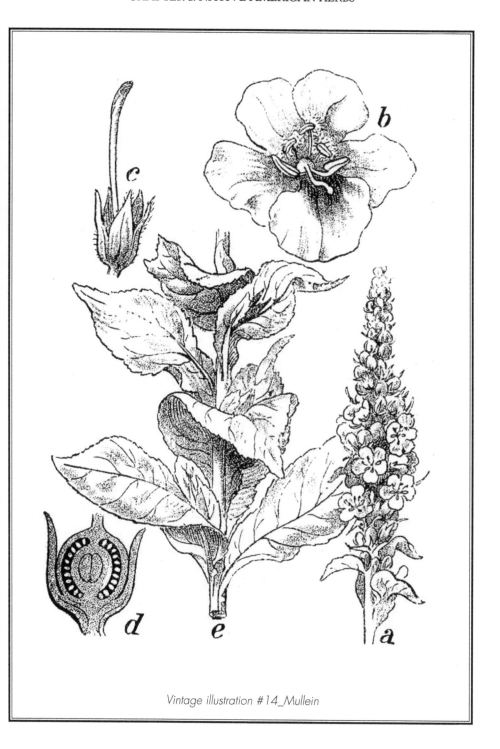

Vintage illustration #14_Mullein

2.28. MAGNOLIA - *Magnolia Grandiflora*

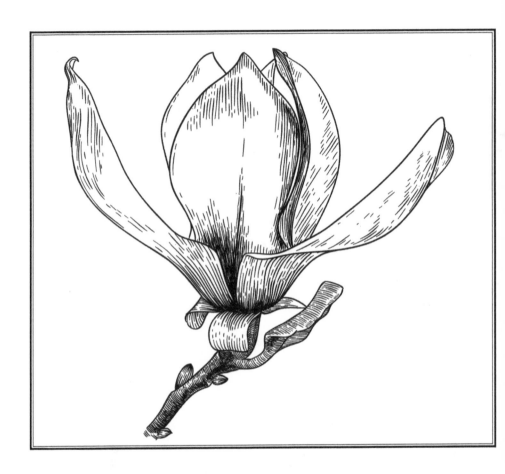

Family: *Magnoliaceae*

Common Names: Beaver Tree, Xin Ye Hua, Xin Yi Hua.

Features: Magnolia is a plant. People use the bark and flower buds to make Medicine.

Uses: For weight loss, stomach disorders, constipation, inflammation, anxiety, stress, depression, flu, headache, stroke, and asthma, magnolia is used.

For stuffy nose, runny nose, common cold, sinus discomfort, hay fever, headache, and dark facial spots, Magnolia flower bud is used.

For toothaches, certain individuals add magnolia flower buds directly to the gums.

Magnolia flower bud extract is used as a skin whitener in rub-on skin care products and to reduce or mitigate skin inflammation caused by the other components.

Magnolia bark is an ingredient of traditional Chinese and Japanese (Kampo) medicine of Hange-koboku-to, which consists of 5 plant extracts, and in Saiboku-to, which consists of 10 plant extracts. To relieve discomfort and nervous stress and to enhance sleep, these extracts are used. Some scholars claim that what makes these drugs work is honokiol, a compound in magnolia bark.

Magnolia appears to have behaviour in animals that decreases fear. It could also increase the body 's development of steroids to combat asthma. Both the magnolia study was in labs.

Sleepiness and drowsiness may be caused by alcohol. Sleepiness and drowsiness may also be caused by Magnolia bark. It could induce too much sleepiness to take large quantities of magnolia bark along with alcohol.

Dose: The adequate dose of magnolia depends on a variety of considerations, such as age, fitness and some other circumstances of the patient. There is not adequate clinical evidence available at this time to establish a reasonable range of doses for magnolia. Bear in mind that not always are natural products inherently healthy and dosages may be essential. Be sure to follow the required product label guidelines and contact the pharmacist or doctor or other healthcare provider before using them.

2.29. NETTLE - *Urtica Dioica*

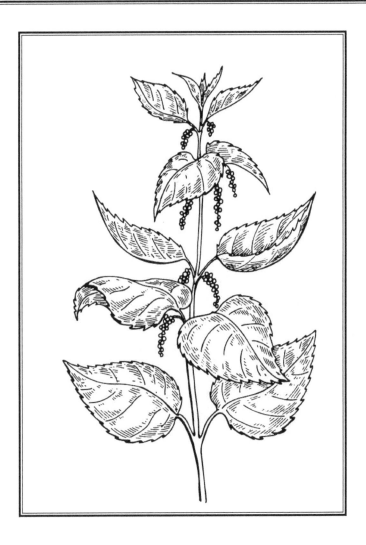

Family: *Urticaceae*

Common Names: Bichu, Common Nettle, Graine d'Ortie, Feuille d'Ortie, Urticae Radix.

Medicinal Part: Stinging nettle is a plant. The above-ground parts and roots are utilized as Medicine.

Uses: For osteoarthritis and diabetes, the Stinging Nettle is used. It is often used for infections of the urinary tract (UTIs), kidney stones, swollen prostate gland, muscle discomfort, among other disorders. However, to confirm these applications, there is no strong scientific research.

Diabetes. In persons with type II diabetes, having stinging nettle leaf prep for 8 to 12 weeks tends to decrease blood sugar.

Osteoarthritis. In individuals with osteoarthritis, having stinging nettle leaf prep by mouth or applying them to the skin can relieve discomfort. The need for pain killers could also be minimized by having stinging nettle leaf prep by mouth. Ingredients that could minimize inflammation and improve urinary output are found in Stinging nettle.

Interactions: With stinging nettle Lithium Interacts. Diabetes medicines (Antidiabetic drugs) interact with stinging nettle. High blood pressure medications (antihypertensive drugs) interact with stinging nettle. The interaction of sedative drugs (CNS depressants) with stinging nettle. The interaction of Warfarin (Coumadin) with stinging nettle

Dose: Scientific research has tested the following doses (for adults):

For diabetes: for 12 weeks, stinging nettle 500 mg leaf extract was taken three times every day by mouth. For 8 weeks, 3.3 g of stinging nettle leaf was also taken three times every day. Also used was a mixed formula comprising stinging nettle 200 mg, milk thistle 200 mg, and frankincense 200 mg given three times a day for three months.

For osteoarthritis: daily use of crude stinging nettle leaf 9 g. An infusion having stinging nettle leaf 5 mg and diclofenac 50 mg every day for 14 days was also taken. For 12 weeks, a particular combination product (medAgil Gesundheitsgesellschaft mbH, Rosaxan) comprising stinging nettle, devil's claw, rosehip, and Vit D was taken by mouth at 40 mL daily was used.

For osteoarthritis, fresh stinging nettle leaves were applied to damaged joints once a day for 30 seconds for one week. For 2 weeks, a particular cream comprising leaf extract of stinging nettle was also used twice every day.

Caution: Pregnancy/breastfeeding, diabetes, and low blood pressure: people with renal issues must use it with caution.

2.30. OREGON GRAPE - *Mahonia Aquifolium*

Family: *Berberidaceae*

Common Names: Holly-leaf barberry, Oregon grape holly, mountain grape, Oregon barberry, blue barberry, Mahonia.

Features: It is a therapeutic herb. Much before the Europeans and other settlers started moving in. The plant has also been used for appetite enhancement in indigenous societies. Today, it is widely used as a replacement for goldenseal, which has similar antimicrobial properties and is now known to be an endangered species owing to over-harvesting.

Medicinal part: The roots (golden yellow) of the plant are utilized for its medicinal properties

Uses: Indigenous tribes of America used the Oregon grape for several illnesses, including fever, jaundice, arthritis, diarrhoea, among other illnesses.

The Oregon grape root has been used to cure numerous illnesses, including colds, flu, hepatitis, herpes, syphilis, upset stomach, tumours, skin conditions, yeast infections, and much more, as herbal medication.

The usage of Oregon grape has been touted by herbalists, saying it successfully stimulates liver activity, cures illnesses, and improves digestive health.

In patients with insulin intolerance, it has been found to reduce blood sugar. It has cholesterol-lowering properties as well.

Oregon Grape is considered to have antifungal and antibacterial effects as an alkaloid derivative of several herbs, including barberry, goldenseal, and other plants. It is known that alkaloids help in battling different kinds of infections. It has been used to relieve problems such as diarrhoea, persistent candidiasis, and more.

In a skin disease called psoriasis, Oregon grape is often known to reduce the immature skin cells overproduction and decrease inflammation.

Interactions: Some drugs can interact with the Oregon grape but might conflict with the body's ability to break down certain forms of liver medications.

Examples of drugs with which Oregon grape should not be taken include:

- Cyclosporine (Neoral, Sandimmune)

- Doxycycline
- Tetracycline
- Any medications that are changed by the liver

Dose: It has been used as a tea widely by boiling few teaspoons (5 to 15 g) of chopped roots in two cups (500 millilitres) of water for 15 mins, then cooling & straining the mixture

Though further tests are required to ensure Oregon grape ingestion protection, herbalists suggest that no more than three cups (750 ml) of tea should be drunk every day.

It is used as a tincture, an alcohol-based herbal blend, supplied at 1/2 - 3/4 teaspoon (3 millilitres) doses and taken per day three times.

A particular mixture of 10 percent extract cream of Oregon grape bark is commercially manufactured as a topical psoriasis cream by a company called Relieva, to be applied to the infected region (around 2 months) of the skin two-three times per day. Often available are creams with a 10 percent Oregon grape root tincture.

Caution: Some drugs can interact with the Oregon grape but might conflict with the body's ability to break down certain forms of liver medications.

Examples of drugs with which Oregon grape should not be taken include: Cyclosporine (Neoral, Sandimmune)' Doxycycline, Tetracycline. Any medications that are changed by the liver.

2.31. PRIMROSE (EVENING) - Oenothera Biennis

Family: *Onagraceae*

Common Names: Aceite de Onagra, Cis-Linoleic Acid, Acide Cis-linoléique,EPO, Evening Primrose, Primrose Oil, Scabish, Sun Drop.

Features: A plant common to South and North America is the evening primrose. It is also rising all over Europe and Asia (parts). It has yellow colour flowers that open at sunset and shut during the day.

Medicinal Part: The seeds oil of evening primrose are utilized.

Uses: For premenstrual syndrome (PMS), menopausal symptoms, swelling, arthritis, and other disorders, evening primrose is used, but no good clinical data is there to justify its use.

Evening primrose oil is also used in foods as an essential fatty acids source.

In the production sector, evening primrose oil is being used in cosmetics and soaps. Evening primrose used to be licensed in Britain to relieve eczema and breast discomfort. The MCA (Medicines Control Agency), the British counterpart to the FDA, has revoked licenses for evening primrose drugs sold for these applications as prescription drugs.

Damage to nerves induced by diabetes. The study suggests that the regular consumption of evening primrose oil for 6 to 12 months enhances the effects of diabetes-induced nerve injury. Osteoporosis. In elderly people with osteoporosis, having evening primrose oil with calcium and fish oil reduces bone loss and improves bone density. There are "fatty acids" in evening primrose oil. Certain women experiencing breast pain do not have large enough amounts of these "fatty acids." Fatty acids often tend to help alleviate inflammation associated with disorders like arthritis and eczema.

Interactions: Antiplatelet/Anticoagulant drugs Medications that delay blood clotting interfere with evening primrose oil.

Anaesthesia medications used during the surgery interacts with the evening primrose oil.phenothiazines interact with the evening primrose oil.

Dose: For Breast pain: 3 to 4 g daily.

2.32. PURSLANE - *Portulaca Oleracea*

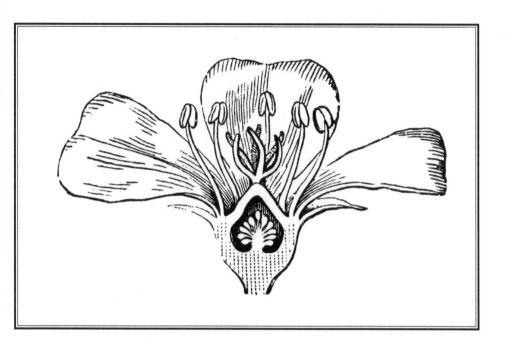

Family: *Portulacaceae*

Common Names: Ma Chi Xian, Garden (common) purslane, Munyeroo, Portulaca, Pourpier, Purslane, Pigweed, Rigla, Sormai

Uses: It is used as fatty acid (omega 3) vegetable source and is rich in minerals and vitamins. It has a pronounced antioxidant function. Roles are indicated in type II diabetes, oral lichen planus asthma, and uterine bleeding, but few and complex clinical trials are, in fact.

Dose: For dosage recommendations, few clinical trials are available; however, 180-milligram purslane extract per day has been tested in diabetic patients, & powdered seeds were taken at 1-30 grams daily in doses divided, also ethanol & aqueous purslane extracts. For a number of indications, traditional Chinese medicine guidelines have been recorded for 9 - 15 grams of dried aerial pieces and 10 - 30 g of fresh herbs. Around 300 - 400 mg, alpha-linolenic acid produces one hundred g of purslane leaves.

2.33. PASSIONFLOWER - *Passiflora Incarnata*

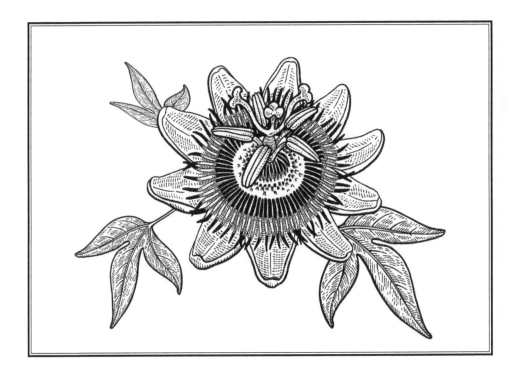

Family: *Passifloraceae*

Common Names: Apricot Vine, Wild Passionflower, Water Lemon.

Uses: Some evidence suggests that taking flowers of passion by mouth will decrease anxiety symptoms. It could potentially function as well as other prescription drugs.

Anxiousness before surgery. Some studies show that when taken 30-90 minutes prior to surgery, taking passionflower by mouth can decrease anxiety before surgery. It may potentially function as well as any other pre-operative anxiety medications, such as melatonin or midazolam.

Interactions: Sedative drugs (CNS depressants) are associated with passionflower.

Sleepiness and drowsiness can be caused by the passionflower. Sedatives are called drugs that induce sleepiness. It might induce too much sleepiness to take passion-flower along with sedative drugs.

Pentobarbital (Nembutal), phenobarbital (Luminal), secobarbital (Seconal), clonazepam (Klonopin), lorazepam (Ativan), zolpidem (Ambien) and others are used in some sedative medicines.

Dose: Clinical research has tested the following doses.

For Adults by mouth. For 2-8 weeks, capsules containing 400 mg of passion flow-er extract were used twice daily for anxiety. In addition, 45 drops of passion flow-er liquid extract were used every day for up to one month.

20 drops of a particular passionflower extract taken the night before surgery and 90 minutes before the beginning of surgery were used to alleviate anxiety before surgery. Tablets of this medication were also taken at a dosage of 500 mg 90 min-utes before the start of the procedure. Passionflower 260 mg taken 30 minutes prior to dental surgery, or 1000 mg of passionflower taken one hour prior to sur-gery. Also, 30 minutes prior to surgery, 5 mL of syrup containing 700 mg of pas-sionflower extract (Passiflora syrup by Sandoz) was taken.

2.34. RED CLOVER - *Trifolium Pratense*

Family: *Legumes*

Common Names: Beebread, Clovone, Cow Clover, Daidzein, Genistein, Isoflavone, Meadow Clover

Features: The red clover is a seedling. The blossoms are used to manufacture medicine. Red clover is prescribed for menopausal complications, frail and delicate muscles, elevated cholesterol levels, and many other disorders, but no good clinical data is sufficient to support these applications. Red clover is used as a flavouring component in meats and drinks. Red clover contains molecules which are similar to the hormone estrogen, or phytoestrogens.

Uses: Enlarged (benign prostatic hyperplasia or BPH) prostate. Any early literature shows that some effects of an enlarged prostate may be relieved by red clover supplements. It tends to minimise urination at night.

There is some early evidence that red clover could help alleviate the discomfort and tenderness of cyclic breast pain.

Menopausal signs. Most tests indicate that taking red clover by mouth would not alleviate symptoms such as hot flashes for up to a year. But some evidence suggests that taking a particular red clover substance (Promensil, Novogen) could decrease the occurrence of hot flashes. Some studies show that the use of red clover can improve vaginal dryness. Other study has also found that red clover can enhance menopausal psychiatric symptoms, such as depression and anxiety. Yet not all review approves.

Possibly ineffective for poor and brittle (osteoporosis) bones. The majority of evidence indicates that the frequent use of red clover does not increase bone density in women.

Insufficient evidence for baldness in male-pattern (androgenic alopecia). Early research suggests that in individuals with hair loss, applying a combination product containing red clover flower extract may improve hair growth.

Large serum levels (hyperlipidaemia) of cholesterol or other fats (lipids). Most evidence suggests that in women who have significantly elevated cholesterol lev

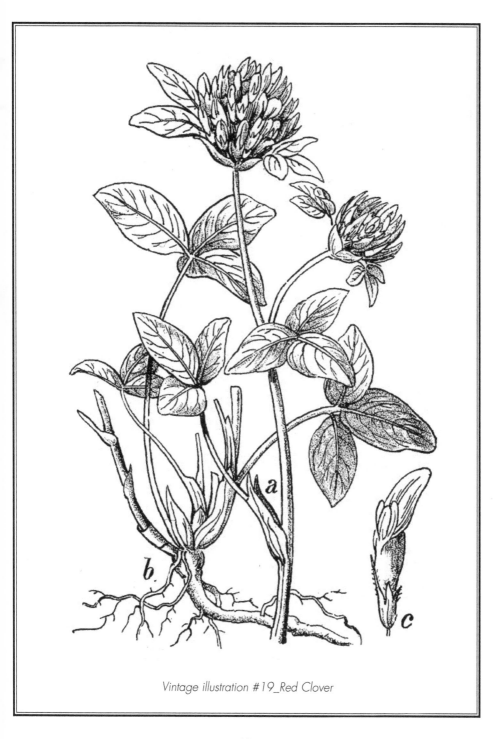

Vintage illustration #19_Red Clover

els, taking red clover extracts by mouth for 3 months to a year does not decrease low-density lipoprotein (LDL or "bad") cholesterol or raise high-density lipoprotein (HDL or "good") cholesterol levels.

More evidence is needed to rate red clover for these uses: Asthma, eczema (atopic dermatitis), breast cancer,

swelling (inflammation) of the main airways in the lung (bronchitis), burns, cough, indigestion (dyspepsia), cancer of the lining of the uterus (endometrial cancer), premenstrual syndrome (PMS), sexually transmitted diseases (STDs), scaly, itchy skin (psoriasis), whooping cough (pertussis), wound healing.

When applied in therapeutic quantities to the skin, red clover is probably healthy.

Dose: The required dosage of red clover depends on a variety of variables, such as age, weight, and some other factors of the user. There is not adequate clinical evidence at this time to establish the optimal range of doses for red clover. Bear in mind that not always are natural products inherently healthy and dosages may be essential. Be sure to follow the required product label guidelines and contact the pharmacist or doctor or other healthcare provider before using them.

Interactions: Moderate interaction.

Medications changed by the liver (Cytochrome P450 2C19 (CYP2C19) substrates) interacts with Red Clover. Some medications are changed and broken down by the liver. Red clover might decrease how quickly the liver breaks down some medications. Taking red clover along with some medications that are broken down by the liver can increase the effects and side effects of some medications. Before taking red clover, talk to your healthcare provider if you take any medications that are changed by the liver. Some medications that are changed by the liver include omeprazole (Prilosec), lansoprazole (Prevacid), and pantoprazole (Protonix); diazepam (Valium); carisoprodol (Soma); nelfinavir (Viracept); and others.

Birth control pills (Contraceptive drugs) interacts with red Clover. Some birth control pills contain estrogen. Red clover might have some of the same effects as estrogen. But red clover isn't as strong as the estrogen in birth control pills. Taking red clover along with birth control pills might decrease the effectiveness of birth control pills. If you take birth control pills along with red clover, use an additional form of birth control such as a condom.

Some birth control pills include ethinyl estradiol and levonorgestrel (Triphas-il), ethinyl estradiol and norethindrone (Ortho-Novum 1/35, Ortho-Novum 7/7/7), and others.

Estrogens interacts with Red Clover. Large amounts of red clover might have some of the same effects as estrogen. But red clover isn't as strong as estrogen pills. Taking red clover along with estrogen pills might decrease the effects of estrogen pills. Some estrogen pills include conjugated equine estrogens (Premarin), ethinyl estradiol, estradiol, and others.

Medications changed by the liver (Cytochrome P450 1A2 (CYP1A2) substrates) interacts with Red Clover. Some medications are changed and broken down by the liver. Red clover might decrease how quickly the liver breaks down some medications. Taking red clover along with some medications that are broken down by the liver can increase the effects and side effects of some medications. Before taking red clover, talk to your healthcare provider if you take any medications that are changed by the liver. Some medications that are changed by the liver include amitriptyline (Elavil), haloperidol (Haldol), ondansetron (Zofran), propranolol (Inderal), theophylline (Theo-Dur, others), verapamil (Calan, Isoptin, others), and others.

Caution: For most people, red clover is likely harmless when consumed by mouth in the proportions found in food. It is probably healthy in therapeutic quantities when used. In certain women, red clover can cause rashes, muscle pain, fever, nausea, and vaginal bleeding (spotting).
Be cautious with this combination.
Pregnancy and breast-feeding. When eaten by mouth in concentrations typically found in food, red clover is possibly healthy. When used in therapeutic quantities, though, it is possibly dangerous. During pregnancy or breast-feeding, red clover behaves like oestrogen and could disrupt major hormone balances. Using it not.
Bleeding disorders. The risk of bleeding may be raised by red clover. Stop massive numbers and use them with caution.
Hormone-sensitive disorders such as cancer of the breast, cancer of the prostate, cancer of the ovary, endometriosis, or fibroids of the prostate: Red clover may

function like estrogen. Don't use red clover if you have some disorder that could be made worse by estrogen.

Protein S deficiency. Individuals with a deficiency in protein S have an elevated chance in blood clots developing. There is some doubt that in these individuals, red clover may increase the risk of clot formation because it has some of the effects of estrogen. If you have protein S deficiency, don't use the red clover.

Surgery: Red clover could delay coagulation of blood. During and after surgery, it may increase the risk of bleeding. Avoid taking the red clover at least 2 weeks before the surgery is scheduled.

2.35. SASSAFRAS - *Sassafras Albidum*

Family: *Lauraceae*

Common Names: Ague Tree, Cinnamon Wood, Bois de Cannelle, Common Sassafras, Saxifrax.

Medicinal Part: To produce medicine, root bark is used.

Uses: despite significant safety issues, there are numerous situations where people use sassafras, but no good empirical data exists to justify these uses.

In the past, sassafras was used in cocktails and sweets to spice root beer. It was used as tea, too. Sassafras tea, though, contains a lot of safrole, the chemical that makes it toxic in sassafras. Around 200 mg of safrole contains one cup of tea made with 2.5 grammes of sassafras. This is about 4.5 times the dosage that experts consider to be lethal. So in 1976, the US Food and Drug Administration (FDA) ruled that it was no longer possible to market sassafras as sassafras tea.

Interactions:

Sedative drugs (CNS depressants) associate with Sassafras Clonazepam (Klonopin), lorazepam (Ativan), phenobarbital (Donnatal), zolpidem (Ambien) among some are some of the sedative drugs.

Dose: A variety of factors, such as the age of the patient, fitness, and many other conditions, depend on the required dose of sassafras. There is no clinical evidence at this stage to establish an acceptable range of doses for sassafras. Bear in mind that not always are natural products inherently healthy and dosages may be essential. Be sure to follow the required product label guidelines and contact the pharmacist or doctor or other healthcare provider before using them.

2.36. SKULLCUP - *Scutellaria Lateriflora*

Family: *Lamiaceae*

Common Names: American Skullcap, Blue Skullcap, Blue Pimpernel, Escutelaria,

Features: It is a flowering perennial plant native to North America used for centuries by Native Americans to treat menstrual disorders, nervousness, and digestive and kidney problems. The name skullcap refers to the flower's resemblance to helmets worn by European soldiers. The above ground parts are used to make Medicine.

Uses: Skullcap is used for stroke-induced trouble sleeping (insomnia), nausea, stroke, and paralysis. It is also used for fever, elevated cholesterol, arterial hardening, rabies, seizures, nervous stress, asthma, skin infections, acne, premenstrual dysphoric disorder (PMDD), and spasms, a significant type of premenstrual syndrome.

Products from Skullcap are not necessarily what the labels say. In skullcap products, the plants germander and teucrium are often undesired and unlabeled ingredients. Scuttelaria lateriflora, the species of skullcap that has been researched for medical use, can also be purchased, but the substance may instead contain a different species of skullcap. Western Skullcap (Scuttelaria canescens), Southern Skullcap (Scutellaria cordifolia) or Marsh Skullcap (Scutellaria galericulatum) are the species most frequently displaced. There are various molecules in these animals, but they are not considered synonymous. It is assumed that the chemicals in the skullcap cause sedation (drowsiness).

Interaction: Interaction with sedative drugs (CNS depressants). Sleepiness and drowsiness can be caused by the skullcap. Sedatives are called drugs that induce sleepiness. It might induce too much sleepiness to take skullcap along with sedative drugs.

Benzodiazepines, pentobarbital (Nembutal), phenobarbital (Luminal), secobarbital (Seconal), thiopental (Pentothal), fentanyl (Duragesic, Sublimaze), morphine, propofol (Diprivan), among some are found in certain sedative medicines.

Dose: The acceptable skullcap dosage depends on a variety of variables, such as age, weight, and many other circumstances of the patient. There is not sufficiently clinical evidence at this time to establish an acceptable range of skullcap doses. Bear in mind that not always are natural products inherently healthy and dosages may be essential. Before using it, be sure to follow relevant guidelines on product packaging and contact your pharmacist or doctor or other healthcare professional.

Caution: Whether you are pregnant or breastfeeding, there is insufficient credible knowledge on the comfort of the skullcap. Stay on the safe side to prevent being seen.

The central nervous system can be slowed down by a skullcap. Healthcare providers fear that this impact may be exacerbated by anaesthesia and other drugs before and during surgery. Avoid taking the skullcap at least 2 weeks before the surgery is set.

2.37 TURKEY CORN - *Dicentra Canadensis*

Family:

Common Names: Dicentra cucullaria, Bleeding Heart.

Features: It originates in Central America's Andean zone. It is among the most essential human and animal cereals and is cultivated for forage and grain.

Medicinal Part: fleshy root (tuber)

Uses: For stomach disorders, urinary tract infections, and skin rashes, people take turkey corn for menstrual conditions. By increasing the urine output, turkey corn may help the body get rid of the extra fluids.

Interaction: with Turkey Corn, lithium interacts.

Dose: The suitable dose of turkey maize depends on many aspects, such as the age, weight, and several other factors of the user. There is no research evidence at this point to establish an acceptable number of doses for it.

Caution: It is better to avoid using turkey maize, especially if you're pregnant/breastfeeding.
Turkey maize might have an impact like a "diuretic" or a water pill. Taking turkey maize could decrease how much lithium gets out of the body. This could raise the amount of lithium and contribute to significant side effects.

2.38. VALERIAN - *Valeriana Officinalis*

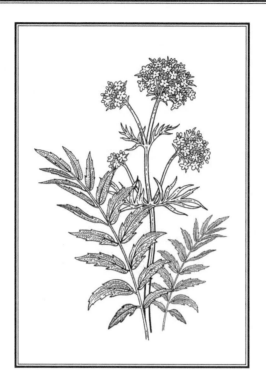

Family: *Valerianaceae*

Common Names: Amantilla, All-Heal, Belgium Valerian, Baldrian, Baldrian-wurzel, Common Valerian

Features: It is originally from Europe and Asia (some parts) but is now rising in North America.

For sleep disorders, particularly insomnia (inability to sleep), Valerian is more widely used. Valerian is often used orally for psychological stress and anxiety.

In processing, valerian extracts and oil are used as flavourings in foods and drinks.

Medicinal Part: Root.

Uses: Insomnia. Although there is some contradictory evidence, most studies suggest that taking Valerian will decrease by around 15 to 20 mins the period it takes to fall asleep. Often, Valerian appears to boost the quality of sleep. Valerian extract doses of 400 to 900 mg taken up to 2 hrs prior to sleep appear to perform best. Before an impact is apparent, consistent usage for many days, perhaps up to one month, can be required. Some reports indicate that Valerian can help enhance sleep when mixed with other herbs, like lemon and balm hops. Valerian can also boost the standard of sleep of persons who refrain from the usage of sleeping tablets. However, some evidence shows that Valerian doesn't really cure insomnia as easily as "sleeping tablets."

Menopausal symptoms. Research suggests that in postmenopausal women, taking 675 to 1060 mg of valerian root every day for eight weeks will reduce the frequency and intensity of hot flashes.

Valerian appears to be working on the brain & nervous system as a sedative.

When administered by mouth regularly for 4 to 8 weeks, Valerian is safe for kids.

Interactions: Liver-changed drugs (substrates of Cytochrome P450 3A4 (CYP3A4)) interact with Valerian.

Such liver-changed drugs include lovastatin (Mevacor), itraconazole (Sporanox), ketoconazole (Nizoral), triazolam (Halcion), fexofenadine (Allegra), and many more.

Dose: Insomnia. 400-900 mg of valerian extract for around six weeks before bedtime, or 120 mg of valerian extract, lemon balm extract 80 mg for up to 30 days or up to 30 days before bedtime.

374 of 500 mg valerian extract + 83.8 to 120 mg hop extract for 2 to 4 weeks before bedtime, or 300 mg valerian extract, passionflower extract 80 mg, and 30 mg of hop extract for up to two weeks before bedtime. Take Valerian 30 mins to 2 hours until bedtime.

For menopause symptoms. For eight weeks, 225 mg ground valerian root was taken three times every day. Even for eight weeks, 530 mg valerian root extract was taken twice every day.

Caution: Inadequate knowledge is available about the protection of Valerian during pregnancy/breastfeeding. For most adults, Valerian is SAFE when consumed by mouth and used in short-term medicinal doses. It is not clear regarding the efficacy of long-term usage.

2.39. WORMWOOD - *Artemisia Absinthium*

Family: *Asteraceae*

Common names: Absinthe, Absinth, Absinthii Herba, Absinthe Suisse, Absinthites, Absinthium.

Medicinal Part: The plant above-ground parts and oil are used.

Uses: It is used for numerous disorders of digestion, such as lack of appetite, gastrointestinal upset, intestinal spasms, and disease of the gall bladder. It is also used to treat the liver's illness, depression, body pain, memory loss, worm infections, and fever, improve sexual desire, induce sweating, and as a tonic. For Crohn's disease and a kidney dysfunction termed IgA nephropathy, wormwood is used. Wormwood oil is often used to enhance the imagination, improve sexual desire, and for digestive disorders.

For osteoarthritis (OA), and for curing wounds and bug bites, certain people apply it directly to the body. To relieve pain, its oil is used as a counterirritant.

When consumed by mouth, wormwood is Harmless in the concentrations typically used in food and drinks, including vermouth and bitters, as long as these items are thujone-free.

Dose: The required dosage of wormwood depends on a number of variables, such as age, fitness, and some other factors of the user. There is not adequate clinical evidence at this point to establish the optimal doses range for wormwood.

Interactions: Medications used to stop Anticonvulsants (seizures) interact with Wormwood

Caution: When ingested by mouth during pregnancy, wormwood is Possibly Unhealthy in concentrations greater than typically present in food. Kidney problems: Taking wormwood oil can induce failure of the kidneys.

Epilepsy and seizure disorders: Wormwood includes thujone, which may induce seizures. There is fear that in people who are vulnerable to them, wormwood may make seizures more probable.

2.40. WITCH HAZEL - *Hamamelis Virginiana*

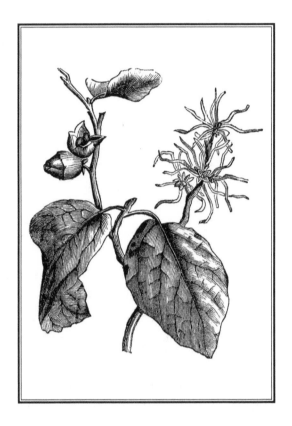

Family: *Hamamelidaceae*

Common Names: Café du Diable, Avellano de Bruja, Hamamelis, Hamamélis de Virginie, Hamamélis, Hamamelis virginiana, Hazel,

Features: It is a deciduous tree or shrub native to North America, and is now planted in Europe and Asia as well. The shrub can reach a height of 4.6 m (15 ft). In the autumn, it flowers, producing bright yellow flowers. Medicine is used to make the leaves, bark, and twigs. You will see a substance (Hamamelis water, purified witch hazel extract) called witch hazel water. It is a solvent distilled from witch hazel's dried stems, bark, and partly dormant twigs.

Witch hazel leaf extract, bark extract, and witch hazel water are used as astringents in processing to tighten the flesh. In certain drugs, they are often used to give certain items the potential to slow down or avoid bleeding. Insect bites, stings, teething, haemorrhoids, swelling, irritations, and mild discomfort are handled with these drugs.

Uses: The application of witch hazel water to the skin can help to temporarily alleviate haemorrhoids and other anal disorders from scratching, inflammation, pain, and burning.

Mild bleeds. The application to the skin of witch hazel bark, herb, or water eliminates moderate bleeding.

Inflammation of the skin. It appears that adding witch hazel cream relieves moderate skin inflammation, but not hydrocortisone as well. Other evidence suggests that the application to the skin of a particular witch hazel ointment (Hametum) tends to relieve signs of skin damage or sore skin as effectively as a childhood dexpanthenol ointment.

Witch hazel contains tannins called chemicals. Witch hazel can help minimise bleeding, help heal damaged skin, and kill bacteria when added directly to the skin.

Kids: Witch hazel, when added directly to the eyes, is likely healthy for kids.

Dose: Clinical research has tested the following doses.

For skin irritation in adults: A 10 percent witch hazel water after-sun lotion was used.

For skin irritation in children aged 2-11 years. An ointment containing witch hazel was applied multiple times a day.

Applied to the rectum. Witch hazel water was administered up to 6 times a day or after a bowel movement for scratching and pain associated with haemorrhoids and other anal disorders. Suppositories were implanted 1-3 times a day into the anus.

Caution: Witch hazel, when actually added to the skin, is LIKELY healthy for most adults. It might cause mild skin irritation in some individuals.

CONCLUSION

The Native American belief in the interconnectedness of human beings and nature is difficult to explain. As ancestors, all part of one large and at least theoretically prosperous family, they looked at all living things, as well as some physical facets of nature, such as rivers, mountains, and climates. We share our breath with everyone that is obvious, writes Native American psychotherapist Robert Blackwolf Jones, the deer, fox, hawk, lizard, tree and shark. The Native American philosopher Chief Seattle shares a similar sentiment, writing: "Man did not weave the web of life, he is merely a thread in it, so that whatever he does to the web, he does to himself."

The Native Americans claimed that a poor interaction with some facets of nature also induced illness. While there were clear explanations for certain forms of injury, such as snake bites and burns, it was difficult to describe internal diseases. The Native Americans thought that the angry spirits of animals, who took vengeance for insults they got in childhood, were more likely to cause "invisible" diseases. "An animal ghost will cause problems if reverence is not given to the body after it has been murdered," according to historian William Corlett. Since Native Americans assumed that humans and nature were closely connected, nearly any thought or behaviour might have negative effects if it displayed contempt for nature. For instance, spitting on a fire could rage the spirits and result in disease.

Nature, of course, has not always been regarded with apprehension. Much as when they were angry, the spirits of animals and other facets of nature could be dangerous, they might also be beneficial when they were happy. For one, the Native Americans believed that herbs and even animals' organs were full of enormous healing powers. During their various curing rituals, they also called on the spirits of animals for help. It was believed that various species had special characteristics and qualities, such as cunning, intellect, and courage. During healing rituals, Native Americans may call for individual animal spirits, asking each in return to share their special gifts with the person being healed. Still, of course, doctors are unlikely to consider calling on the spirits of eagles and bears to regulate blood pressure or cure arthritis, but depending on how it is handled, they are very mindful of nature's ability to cure or hurt. For example, prolonged exposure to sunlight can cause cancer, but when the sun is used properly (approximately 15 minutes of everyday exposure), it makes the body produce vitamin D, which is necessary for healthy bones. Nutrients are filled with the foods we consume, such as vitamin A, iron, folate, and sodium are important to life in right quantity; in abundance, all of them can be dangerous. Since the keys to wellbeing are peace and order, who does not benefit from learning a lesson from the Native American people? The way to start is by treating with the highest regard the world around us. "It's time we climbed down from the lonely pedestal we've made for ourselves, according to Robert Blackwolf Jones, and we remember our position alongside our fellow inhabitants."

ABOUT THE AUTHOR

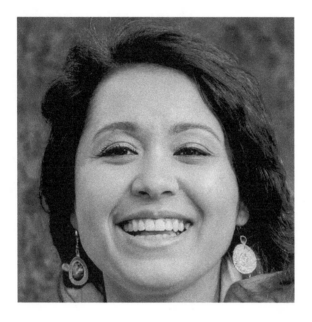

Tamaya Kawisenhawe was born in Santa Barbara and earned her master's degree in botany at Claremont Graduate University (California).

After becoming a naturopathic and acupuncturist, she moved to Portland where she lives with her husband and two daughters. She has worked with medicinal herbs for more than 15 years.

Now, she decides to share and spread her passion and knowledge with others, running seminars all around the country.

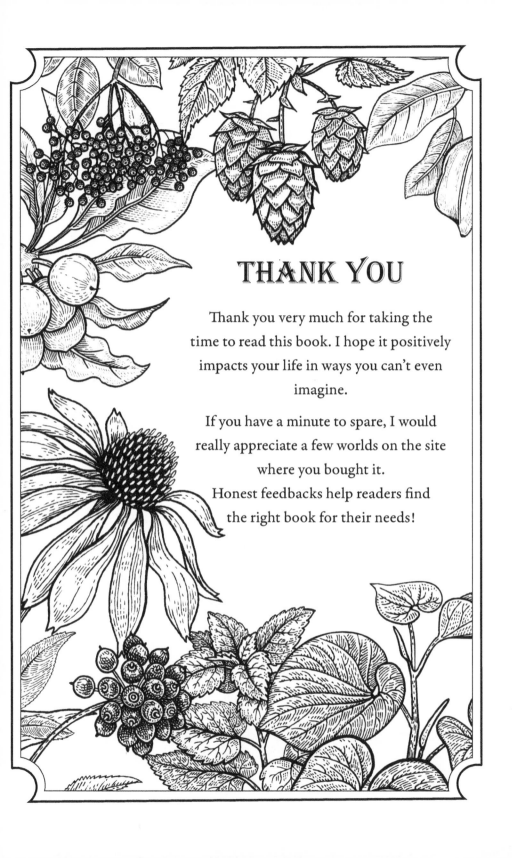

THANK YOU

Thank you very much for taking the time to read this book. I hope it positively impacts your life in ways you can't even imagine.

If you have a minute to spare, I would really appreciate a few worlds on the site where you bought it.
Honest feedbacks help readers find the right book for their needs!

CPSIA information can be obtained
at www.ICGtesting.com
Printed in the USA
BVHW031705050421
604207BV00008B/849

9 781801 112789